BE YE TRANSFORMED

STRATEGIES FOR MIND RENEWAL AND BEHAVIOR CHANGE TO ACHIEVE THE BODY YOU DESIRE

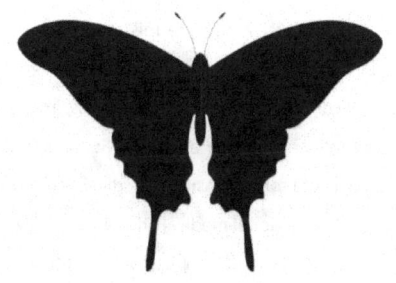

By Tracey Garito Mahaney

Table of Contents

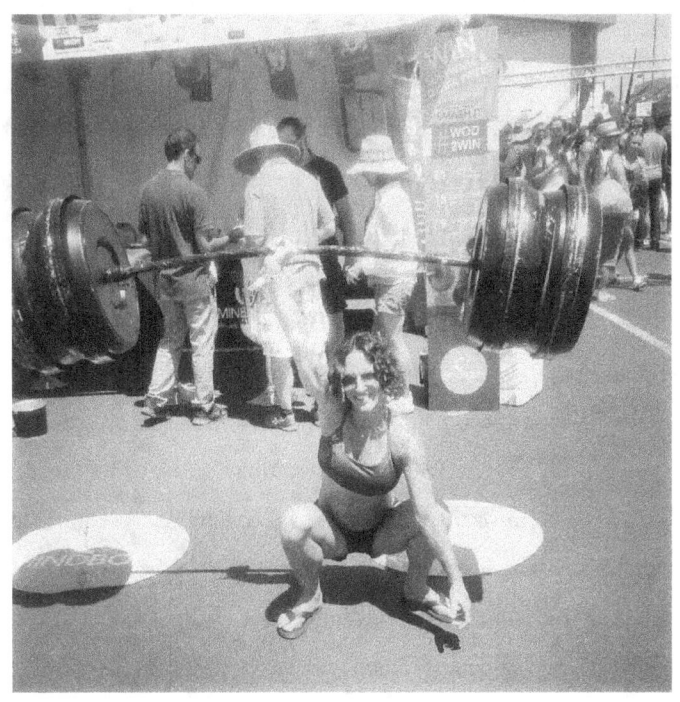

My Story

I have been where you are.

I write this less than two months after my fortieth birthday. In my 40 years I have lived many different diet and exercise programs and I can assure you it has not been a linear process. I have been fat/overweight. I have been through stages of extreme dieting and extreme exercising. I have suffered from disordered eating and starved myself down to 95 pounds. I know what it's like to not want to look in the mirror. I know how it feels to hate being naked. I know how it feels to be so unhappy with your body that you hide it under layers of baggy clothes. I have been where you are. I was constantly researching the latest diet and exercise strategies (and fads) searching desperately for that magic pill. Every time I heard about a new diet I had to try it. You name it I've done it. I was frustrated that no matter how hard I tried I was never able to achieve lasting results.

After every failure (which was often) I always defaulted to the same behavior. And instead of figuring out why I had failed (or rather, what behaviors had failed me), I'd move on to the next extreme diet/exercise strategy hoping this time things would be different.

It took me over twenty years to finally realize that it isn't a one-size-fits-all approach. What works for one person may not work for another. Through research, experience, trial-and-error, self-examination and self-experimentation I have found a sustainable plan that creates real significant lasting results. The truth is there is nothing magical about it. It was just a combination of behaviors that added up to big results.

When I set out to write this book I knew I didn't want it to be just another diet book. If I have learned one thing over the years it's that just knowing what to eat and what not to eat is not enough. The difference between success and failure for me meant a complete shift in my *thinking* and a change in my *behaviors*. My goal is to draw from my experience and share what has worked for me, the specific actions I took, and the behavior change strategies I employed that have allowed transformation to happen and resulted in lasting change. I want to share any details of my journey that may help you reach the same results in your life, even if your path looks slightly different from mine.

My Story

Over the course of my lifetime my diet and exercise programs have changed and evolved. Below is an overview of the chronology.

Stage #1 – The Standard American Diet

Growing up I was always active. As a child I enjoyed playing soccer, tetherball, kick-the-can, and flashlight tag, riding bikes, playing in the dirt and building forts with the other kids in the neighborhood. In middle school and high school I played field hockey. I wasn't coordinated, fast, or athletic enough to be good, so they made me a goalie (No offense to goalies! I've played with some really good ones).

For the first 16 years of my life I ate a conventional diet which consisted of *a lot* of processed foods. The staples included lots of cereal, peanut butter and jelly sandwiches (made with white bread), frozen burritos, Ramen noodles, Pop Tarts, spaghetti and M&Ms – not much different from most kids and teens at the time.

Stage #2 – The Low-Fat Era

Unfortunately my teenage years coincided with the "low-fat era" where the idea was if people just reduced the fat content of their diet they would be improving it. It also happened to be the time that I began to shift my focus to my appearance. It was then that I began to use diet and exercise to control my shape, size and weight rather than for health and enjoyment. I made my diet and exercise reflections of who I was as a person. When I was not what I would consider perfect I deemed myself a failure. My self-worth was based on my appearance, specifically the size and shape of my body. The staples of my diet included still more processed food loaded with additives, preservatives, chemicals, artificial sweeteners and added sugars: dry pasta (seasoned only with salt, pepper and Butter Buds), bagels with Promise Ultra fat-free margarine, "healthy" cereal with skim milk, "lite" bread, soft pretzels, diet soda, Slim Fast, and fat-free Snackwell cookies. (Carbs, carbs, and more carbs). On the rare occasion I would eat chicken but I thought it was too high in fat to consume on a regular basis. As long as I consumed zero fat and stayed under my allotted 800 calories for the day I was okay as far as I was concerned.

I was a very skinny (95 pounds), very hungry (starving), very unhealthy (sick), very sad (depressed) little girl. Every morning, when I opened my eyes, the first thing I thought about was what I would eat that day... and what I wouldn't eat. My self-worth depended on whether I ate foods off of what I referred to as the "good" list or the "bad" list. Each night I'd go to sleep vowing that tomorrow I'd "be better." I counted calories in *everything*... sugarless gum (5 calories), black coffee (5 calories). I knew nothing - and cared little - about the nutritional value of what I was eating. It didn't matter if it was processed, had no expiration date and an unpronounceable ingredients list a mile long. As long as it wouldn't make me "fat," that was all I cared about.   Hunger pains gave me a sense of control. But I had no idea then how out of control I really was.

Flash back to 1990 (my junior year of high school)...A typical day of eating for me:
Breakfast:
1 cup corn flakes cereal (100 calories)

1 cup skim milk (80 calories)

1 packet of Equal Sweetener (5 calories)

1 cup black coffee with artificial sweetener (5 calories)

Snack:

1 granny smith apple (80 calories)

Lunch:

1 cup cooked pasta, dry (175 calories) with salt, pepper & Butter Buds (5 calories)

Snack

1 granny smith apple (80 calories)

Dinner:

1 cup cooked pasta, dry (175 calories) with salt, pepper & Butter Buds (5 calories) OR whatever my mom made... but no more than what would fit on a *small* dinner plate.

Stage #3 – Starvation Diets and Binge Eating

I continued to starve myself until one day my body just rebelled. I remember it as if it were yesterday. It was the day before Thanksgiving 1990. My grandparents were visiting for the holiday and I wanted them to taste the chocolate chip cookies I had made from scratch. As a way to strengthen my willpower, I would often bake cookies and cakes but not allow myself to eat them... and if I could get others around me to eat them it would just prove how strong I really was. I was in awe at how my grandparents were able to enjoy a cookie (or two!) without a second thought. And they didn't even seem to show any guilt, shame or remorse afterwards. It was fascinating. So the thought occurred to me that maybe I could have a cookie... just one. What harm would it do? So I had one. And the flood gates opened. After having several cookies I pulled out a box of Kix cereal and proceeded to consume three bowls. Now this may not seem like a big deal to you, but for a 16 year-old with a messed up self-esteem and a distorted body image that had spent the past six months starving herself down to a "petite" size three, consuming two chocolate chip cookies and three bowls of cereal in one sitting was a VERY big deal. That moment was a turning point for me... and not in a good way. In November my size three Gap jeans hung loosely on my hips. By February, less than three months later, I had gained over 40 pounds and was barely squeezing myself into a size 13/14.

I spent the next several years on a roller coaster ride of starvation diets, binge eating, diet pills, over-exercising, self-destructive, obsessive-compulsive behaviors and lots of therapy. My workout routine was sporadic at best and consisted of mostly cardio. I had no interest in being strong or even healthy for that matter. All that mattered to me was being skinny. It was a nightmare that I wouldn't wish on anyone. You couldn't pay me any amount of money to go back to that period in my life.

Stage #4 – A Gym Rat is Born

By the grace of God, I was introduced to weight training by a friend at around the age of 20 and immediately fell in love with it! I spent my life at the gym. I did forty-five minutes to an hour (or more) of cardio every day and then your traditional body-builder type split routine: chest, shoulders and triceps on day one, back and biceps on day two, legs on day three, one day off and repeat. I read everything I could get my hands on about health, fitness and nutrition.

Then it dawned on me—Why not get certified? So I did....and that's where my personal training journey began, with a basic personal training certification and a position as a trainer at a New York Sports Clubs (NYSC). The more I learned, the more my own workouts evolved. I began adding flexibility, mobility, core, balance, stabilization and power training to my programs. But I still couldn't pull myself away from the long, boring workouts and one-hour long cardio sessions every day. I even had a staff member approach me one day and say, "The treadmill asked if you could please take a day off. It's tired."

In 2000 I completed my first marathon. I was proud of my accomplishment but really I just did it because I thought for sure that the training regime (lots and lots of running) would make me skinny. I continued with my low-fat, high-carb, fat-phobic diet, yet still couldn't manage to get rid of that extra ten pounds of fat I was carrying around. I was baffled.

Stage #5 – The Low-Carb Craze

In the late 1990s and early 2000s came the "low-carb craze" when low carbohydrate diets like The Atkins Diet and other diets with similar principles became the most popular diets in the country. Willing to try anything, I jumped on the bandwagon. It was the first diet I had tried up to that point that "allowed" me to eat meat and fat without (as much) fear. Yet I still found myself on a diet then off a diet then back on a diet... and every Monday was day one.

Stage #6 – Training for Ms. Figure

In 2004 I decided to compete for the title of Ms. Figure. What I put my poor body through in an effort to achieve the level of musculature, leanness and vascularity necessary was nothing short of abuse. My workouts consisted of 45-60 minutes of cardio every morning and another 45-60 minutes of cardio every night along with my regular weight training routine. I began carb cycling, which is an aggressive strategy designed for short-term use. In the most basic format, carb cycling is a planned alteration of carbohydrate intake in order to prevent a fat loss plateau and maintain metabolism along with athletic performance. The staples of my diet included baked chicken, egg whites, "low-carb" pancakes, oatmeal and steamed broccoli. Every three days I was allowed one half-cup of rice with butter and a banana. My training was just a means to an end. I did it all to look a certain way... and to win. I had no visible body fat anywhere on my body. There was visible separation between my muscles and you could see the veins in my forearms, calves and lower abs. My body fat percentage was below average (23% body fat is considered average for women and 18% is considered "athletic." I was down around 15%). All my hard work paid off and in 2004 I won the title NABBA USA Ms. Figure USA! (http://www.nabba.com/resultsjrnat04.cfm). For the first time in my life I actually liked the way my body looked. But to sustain it was pure torture. The thrill of victory was short-lived. When the competition was over I eased up on my insane training and extremely restrictive diet and, naturally, I gained some body fat. Even with the weight gain following the competition, my body composition was still in the "below average" range for women. But when I looked in the mirror I just saw a fat person. I had failed... again.

In that same year I left the "globo gym" world and opened a one-on-one personal training franchise. I finally had "my own place." In addition to working one-on-one with clients, I trained and developed a solid team of trainers. I was running a successful business and helping hundreds of clients reach their health and fitness goals. But I still was not at peace with myself and my body.

Stage #7 – Clean(er) Eating + the Zone

By 2007, after years of research and self-experimentation, I had cleaned up my diet quite a bit. I was making food choices that I believed would not only help me get lean, but that would also make me healthier. My main staples were egg whites, grilled chicken, broiled salmon, steamed vegetables, green salads, fruit, nuts and a small amount of whole grains, dairy and soy products. My cereal / grain consumption was typically in the form of sprouted grain breads, steel cut oats, and, occasionally, brown rice. My dairy / soy consumption was typically in the form of soy milk (with my oatmeal), cottage cheese, and skim lattes. I was also committed to strict adherence to the parameters of Dr. Barry Sears' Zone Diet (http://zonediet.com/) which meant weighing and measuring everything I ate. Thirty percent of my calories came from low-glycemic carbohydrates, forty percent from lean protein, and thirty percent from "good" fat.

Stage #8 – Paleo and CrossFit

In 2009, I was out one night having dinner with my good friend, Karianne – a fellow trainer, and former co-worker at NYSC, whom I respect and admire immensely. She had just gotten back from a CrossFit (http://crossfit.com/) Level 1 Seminar. The excitement and enthusiasm was coming out of her pores! I had heard of CrossFit and had even done an occasional WOD (Workout Of the Day) here and there, but nothing consistent. In addition to talking about CrossFit she also mentioned a way of eating called the Paleolithic Diet – commonly referred to as the caveman or paleo diet – which I had never heard of before (I'll talk more about the details of the Paleo Diet later). For the weeks and months following my dinner with Karianne, her words replayed over and over again in my head. My interest was piqued.

When I first heard about the paleo diet I had some reservations. By that time, my diet was pretty good compared to most people I knew... I was finally healthy and I felt good. At least I thought so. The modifications necessary for me to "go paleo" were relatively small. I couldn't imagine it would make much of a difference. But I was curious enough to give it a try. Boy was I in for a surprise! Within days I noticed a dramatic improvement in my energy levels and sleep quality. I noticed my sinuses were clearer and my skin glowed. Within a week I actually started to notice a change in my body composition (with seemingly little effort). In less than two weeks I stopped craving the foods that at one point I couldn't imagine living without (sugar, grains and starchy carbs). Over the next few weeks my bowel function normalized (Halleluiah!) and I no longer experienced the post-meal bloating and indigestion that I just attributed to overeating. My athletic performance improved – I got measurably faster and stronger. At the age of 35 I was looking, feeling and performing better than I ever had in my life!

That same year I closed my one-on-one personal training studio and became a CrossFit affiliate... transform CrossFit (http://www.transformcrossfit.com/) was born. In June 2009, transform CrossFit opened its doors at 10 North Main Street in Pennington, New Jersey. Since the beginning, we have had three primary goals: 1) to educate our clients and our community on the benefits of CrossFit and Paleolithic Nutrition, 2) to change lives and 3) to pursue excellence.

I started eating paleo (and CrossFitting) in 2009 and have never looked back. Today eating Paleo is just a way of life for me. It's not a diet. It's a lifestyle. I eat enough to sustain energy levels and fuel athletic performance. I can honestly say that I like my body. I'm strong and lean and I like the way my clothes fit. I'm not real big on weighing myself these days but I fit comfortably into a size two! I am never hungry - except on the rare occasion I don't prepare enough food ahead of time.... and when I am hungry, I eat. I never feel deprived. Sure, there are foods that I miss (and, on the rare occasion, I will indulge) but I no longer crave them constantly. When considering my food options for any given meal, my decisions are based on how I will feel thirty minutes after I've finished eating (content vs. full and sluggish) and how it will affect my athletic performance and recovery and, most importantly, my health. My self-worth isn't even a thought because, today, how "good" or "bad" I am has nothing to do with my food choices. My body is not perfect (and that's okay) but I appreciate it for what it can do. I am strong, healthy and happy and I wouldn't trade that for anything.

For the first time in my life, thanks to the paleo diet, I have a healthy relationship with food and my body.

Before discovering CrossFit and paleo, I completed two figure competitions and three marathons, and I can honestly say that, at 40 years-old (the time this was written) I am in the best shape of my life. And the best part is it doesn't just stop at my workouts. It has translated into <u>every</u> area of my life. It has changed the way I feel, the way I look, the way I think. It has given me the courage to step out of my comfort zones and try things that, before, may not have seemed possible.

Step 1 –
Change the Way You Think

I was determined to find a way of eating that worked for me and my body type. But I was so sick of dieting (and failing). I didn't need another diet. I needed a new life plan. I needed a better way of living, not as something I'd do for a few weeks to reach some artificial, short-term goal. What I wanted was complete *transformation*.

If you are reading this I think it's fairly safe to assume that (1) You are not happy with the current state of your health, appearance, and/or level of fitness, (2) You are looking for a way to create significant change with sustainable results that you can maintain for the next five or more years and (3) You recognize that what you've been doing isn't working for you.

Transformation is about growth, new thinking, and permanent change. For me permanent change required a renewal of my thoughts and attitudes – a renewing of my mind. It was no longer about "trying really hard" to avoid certain foods for a specific amount of time, or "will-powering" my way through workouts hoping to achieve a new personal record (PR). *It has been said that the way you think determines the way you feel, and the way you feel determines the way you act (behavior). So if you want to change the way you act (and feel), you have to start by changing the way you think.* For example, I can say, "I want to eat better" or "I want to perform better." But in order to do that I would need to first change the way I *think* about food/nutrition and exercise, which will change the way I *feel* about food/nutrition and exercise, which will change the way I *act.*

I finally realized that if I was going to change anything about my behavior or my emotions I would have to start by changing my thoughts and attitudes. It's about turning *from* something bad, and turning *towards* something good. It's turning from condemnation to acceptance; turning from pessimism to optimism; turning from discouragement to hopefulness; turning from guilt to forgiveness.

For me, this journey has been about changing the way I think about food; changing the way I think about exercise; changing the way I think about my past, my present and my future. At the end of the month I want to be stronger physically, mentally, emotionally, and spiritually. But it doesn't end there. In six months I want to be stronger than I will be a month from now. In one year I want to be stronger than I will be six months from now. But in order for me to achieve those goals I needed start by changing my thinking.

Step 2 –
Change Your Focus

I believe that it is important to set goals. You've heard the acronym S.M.A.R.T. goals. SMART goals are Specific, Measurable, Attainable, Realistic, and Time-bound. Everyone should set SMART goals. An example of a SMART goal is: "I want to take two inches off my waist in 60 days." It's specific and measureable (two inches), it's attainable (assuming you make the appropriate lifestyle changes), it's realistic (as opposed to expecting to lose 10 pounds in one week) and it's time-bound (60 days). Goals give us purpose, something to strive for. But once you have set your goals, I believe that if you want to achieve lasting results it's important to focus on the *process*... not the outcome. For example, if fat loss is a goal, it's important that your focus be on making changes that *allow* fat loss to occur, *not* on numbers on a scale.

Remember, you can't change how you behave (and look and feel) until you change how you think! You must zoom out and look at the bigger picture. You must rid yourself of unwanted behaviors and adopt new ones that would make fat loss possible. Focus not being a size two, getting six pack abs, or losing a certain amount of weight... but rather on what behaviors you need to adopt to achieve that outcome and what thoughts you need to adopt to achieve those behaviors. Without some behavior change strategies any achievement would not be sustainable over time.

I will be open about my flaws and struggles. I don't claim to have all the answers. I will share my experiences - my successes and my failures – but what worked and didn't work for me may not be the same for you. I believe wholeheartedly in a Paleolithic lifestyle but I'm not going to force it on anyone. Before you move forward I encourage you to take a hard, honest look at where you are now (and why), and where you have been and to be brutally honest with yourself about what is and is not working for you. That kind of honesty takes courage.

I think it's a safe assumption that what you have been doing isn't working for you or you probably wouldn't be reading this. It's been said that the most powerful tool in healing is the willingness and open-mindedness to try a new way when what you've been doing is not helping you live as healthily as you could. You know the definition of insanity don't you? Insanity is doing the same thing over and over again and expecting a different result. Explore your options, experiment and find what works for your body type. It's not a one-size-fits-all endeavor. Build an eating plan piece-by-piece that will work for YOU. If you want results that are sustainable, that you can maintain over the long-term, then the plan must fit with who you are and how you live your life.

- Do you want to change your relationship with and attitude towards food for good?
- Do you want to increase awareness of destructive habits, such as: overeating, eating too much of something and not enough

of something else, life revolving around food, eating for fuel and function vs. emotional eating?

- Do you want to identify what your cues/triggers are that stimulate a particular food response (desired or detrimental)?
- Do you want to figure out some strategies specific to your motivational stage, resources, lifestyle and emotional needs that will enable you to maintain substantial, lasting food behavior change?
- Do you want to end the vicious cycle and get rid of those addictive foods that leave you feeling toxic?
- Do you want to reset your taste buds to desire healthier and more natural foods?
- Do you want to eliminate your cravings for starchy, sugary foods?
- Do you want to improve athletic performance?
- Do you want/need accountability, guidance and support?

...then keep reading!

Step 3 –

Take an Honest Inventory

Where Are You?

Before I could get to where I wanted to be, I needed to figure out where I was and *why*. That required me to be brutally honest with myself about the behaviors that had gotten me to the place where I was. I needed to express in a clear and honest way what was working and what wasn't working for me without trying to sugar coat it. I had to take an honest assessment of how certain behaviors were hindering my progress and how my food choices were negatively affecting my health, mood, sleep, athletic performance, body composition, bowel function and energy levels.

Here is my list:

1. I am an emotional eater.
2. I don't have the self-control or the willpower to avoid junk food if it's in my house. Whether it's ice cream, chocolate, cheese, wine or cereal... If it's there I will consume it.
3. When I don't plan and prepare my meals I make poor (usually emotional) food choices.
4. I will finish whatever is on my plate / in front of me. If I don't measure and then portion my food I will continue to (over)eat until my plate is empty.

5. As I get older I find there is less and less I can get away with. My body is not as forgiving as it once was. I must pay careful attention to what and how much I eat.

6. I cannot consume chocolate, grains, dairy products or wine on a regular basis and expect to achieve the body I want.

7. When I make poor food choices I gain body fat. When I gain body fat my self-confidence suffers. This affects all areas of my life.

8. When I make poor food choices I physically feel like crap. When I feel like crap I'm not very motivated to eat well. And the vicious cycle begins...

9. When I make poor food choices my sleep suffers. I have trouble falling asleep and I don't sleep soundly. In the morning I wake up grumpy.

10. When I make poor food choices I don't enjoy my workouts and my athletic performance suffers.

11. When I don't decide ahead of time when my "treats" will occur and what they will be they tend to happen more frequently than they would otherwise.

12. I rationalize poor food choices by telling myself that I eat better than most people I know (as if that makes a difference to my body).

13. I am a perfectionist. I tend to think in black-and-white, all-or-nothing terms.

Take a look at this list of **THE TOP 10 NUTRITIONAL AND DIETARY MISTAKES PEOPLE MAKE** (http://www.primalbody-primalmind.com/top-10-nutritional-mistakes/) by Nora T. Gedgaudas, author of Primal Body – Primal Mind | Beyond the Paleo Diet for Total

Health and a Longer Life (http://www.primalbody-primalmind.com/) and see if any of it sounds familiar….

10) Relying on superficial descriptions such as "natural" or even "organic" to determine whether a food is truly healthy.

9) Relying on the media, your doctor, or even conventional nutritionists/dieticians to provide accurate nutritional information.

8) Believing that junk food "in moderation" is OK.

7) Following "government guidelines" or "The Food Pyramid" for healthy eating.

6) Thinking that being "slim" means you are healthy – using weight as your litmus of "good health."

5) Using vitamins to make up for unhealthy eating habits.

4) Believing that exercise can "make up" for unhealthy eating habits.

3) The belief that "genetics is destiny."

2) The belief that eating healthy means having to give up the enjoyment of food, good flavor, fat, dietary cholesterol, or animal source foods.

1) The belief or assumption that eating a quality diet is too expensive…or too difficult or complicated to maintain.

For more details visit www.primalbody-primalmind.com and read Primal Body – Primal Mind | Beyond the Paleo Diet for Total Health and a Longer Life. (You'd better have your highlighter ready!)

Conduct a Wellness Audit

Answer the questions on this list with the numbers: 0, 1, 2 or 3.

0 = Frequently, 1 = Sometimes, 2 = Rarely, 3 = Never

1. *Do you experience headaches?*
2. *Do you tend to get a cold and/or virus each year?*
3. *Do you have bowel movements less than several times per day?*
4. *Do you experience constipation?*
5. *Do you experience diarrhea?*
6. *Do you experience pain and/or stiffness in your joints or muscles?*
7. *Do you experience itchy and/or watery eyes and nose at certain times of year?*
8. *Do you experience congestion or mucus in your throat?*
9. *Do you get bloated after eating?*
10. *Do you have extra body fat that you cannot seem to lose with exercise and/or diet?*
11. *Do you experience indigestion heartburn, gas, and/or acid stomach?*
12. *Do you have bad breath?*
13. *Do you have body odor?*
14. *Do you crave certain foods, especially starchy, sugary foods?*
15. *Do you have a skin condition such as itchy skin or pimples?*
16. *Do you have low energy levels?*

17. *Do you rely heavily on caffeine for energy?*

18. *Do you experience restless sleep and/or insomnia?*

19. *Do you experience bad moods, sadness, or depression?*

Now add up all of the numbers to figure out your score (Be sure to write it down. You'll need to refer back to it later).

"Before" Photos and Measurements

1. Take a photo of yourself (using a cell phone camera is fine) wearing as little as possible. I realize this part may be difficult, but if you don't take a 'before' photo and you follow through with this program you will be kicking yourself later. Trust me.

2. Using a tape measure, take and record the following measurements:

   - Your hips at the widest part (be sure to keep the tape level).
   - Your waist at the belly button (*not* the narrowest part).

I encourage you to <u>stay off the scale</u> during this process (I'll explain why in Step Seven)...

Step 4 –
Keep a Log

My experience suggests that most people are not very good at estimating how many calories they eat on any given day. Most people, it seems, *think* they eat less than they actually do. That's the scary part. No one gains 30 pounds overnight. It happens gradually over time. It just takes an extra 100 calories here and there. You could easily (mindlessly) eat 100-300 more calories today than you did yesterday and not even realize it. If you consistently eat 300 calories per day more than your body needs, the result would be a two- to three-pound weight gain *each month*! In one year you would be *30 pounds* heavier than you are right now! (It takes an excess of 3500 calories to gain one pound)

Often, in an effort to eat "healthier" and/or lose weight, people will *under eat* which can cause hunger, mood swings, cravings, poor sleep and anxiety. Deprivation diets that restrict our daily calorie intake by 600-800 calories a day are not sustainable over time. They send a "starvation" message to the metabolism telling it to slow down. This slowing of the metabolism is what helped our hunter-gatherer ancestors survive famines. These crash diets only set us up for a binge later so any weight that is lost quickly returns (and then some). Fortunately, making a few *small* behavior changes at a time is relatively easy. With just a few minor adjustments you could easily cut out 200-300 calories a day. Your body won't miss those calories and in one year you would weigh up to 30 pounds less than if you hadn't made any adjustments.

If I had a nickel for every time a client has approached me and said, *"I eat very 'healthy' but I'm just not seeing results "* or,*" I've been following the paleo way of eating for over a month now. I lost a few pounds in the first couple of weeks but I've hit a plateau. I don't understand what's going on."* My first question to them is, "Are you keeping a food log?" The answer almost every time is no. The phrases "eating healthy" or "following the paleo diet" do not give me enough information to be able to help the client.

If you are going to figure out what is and isn't working for you it is of the utmost importance that you be completely honest about what your current diet looks like. The best way to do that is to keep a detailed food log of everything that you eat. So many people are unhealthy and overweight because they have no idea *what* and *how much* they are actually eating or *why* they are eating it. They repeat the same destructive habits and behaviors day after day, week after week, month after month, and year after year, sometimes without even realizing it. **It's important that you start keeping a detailed food log right now BEFORE you start making any dietary changes.** Think of it as a "before" snapshot of your current diet (the one that isn't working for you). It will be helpful to have this to look back at later.

What to Record:

Simply jotting down what you had for breakfast lunch and dinner is not going to be enough if you are looking to produce permanent change. You will need more data than that if you want some clues as to what is and isn't working for you. In *Step Nine – Behavior Change Strategies* we'll talk about identifying your triggers that produce detrimental behaviors (i.e. unconscious eating or consumption of large quantities of certain types of foods) as well as those triggers that produce positive behaviors. The goal is mindfulness. Some important details to record include:

- Detailed food and fluid intake
- Portion size
- Time of day
- Where you are
- Who you are with / Social setting
- Your degree of hunger (i.e. 0 = not hungry, 1 = hungry, 2 = very hungry)
- Your emotional state
- How you feel one hour after eating (physically AND mentally)

There are plenty of online services / applications (many of them FREE) that will give you an automatic breakdown of macronutrients (proteins, carbohydrates and fats), micronutrients (vitamins and minerals), calories, sodium and sugar!

Why Food Logs Work
- They are a great tool for determining how what goes into your body affects body composition, mood, athletic performance, sleep habits, etc.
- They make you more accountable (even more so if you're showing your food log to someone else). I have been keeping a food log

for over five years now. I record everything I eat. Usually no one sees it except me. But it's no coincidence that I eat better (and more mindfully) when I'm keeping one than when I'm not!

- They increase awareness of certain patterns, habits and triggers. Once you're aware of a destructive pattern, you have the power to change it.
- They do not depend on memory.
- Online services or applications provide accurate intake data such as calories, macronutrients and micronutrients.

Tips on Keeping a Food Log

- **Record as you go.** Don't wait until the end of the day to record everything you ate and drank. You are likely to forget something... especially if it's something you wish you hadn't eaten.
- **Schedule it in.** If you are not able to update your log after every meal or snack, pick a time each day when you will update it. Write it on your schedule and treat it just like an appointment.
- **Remember the B.L.T. Rule:** If you bite it, lick it or taste it, it should be recorded! Most of us have good intentions when it comes to nutrition. I can assure you, it isn't that grilled chicken over a green salad with the dressing on the side that is sabotaging your weight loss efforts. Many times it's the mindless eating – picking off the kids' plates, taking a piece of chocolate each time you walk by the candy dish, grabbing a cookie ("just one") because you were hungry and it's all you had time for as you rushed out the door. Those are the things that sometimes add up to several hundred calories at the end of the day (*and* stimulate an insulin

response that sends a message to your body to store fat. More on that later).

- **Focus on portion size**. Most people underestimate how much they eat. Practice using measuring cups and spoons when you're at home until you are able to "eyeball" what a half-cup looks like. I also recommend getting yourself a digital food scale to weigh your protein sources (You can purchase a good one for $20).
- **Be consistent.** Whether you use a notebook, an excel spreadsheet, an app, or a cell phone camera (a photo log) be sure you are using it consistently!
- **Don't skip your indulgent days.** It's especially important to write on days you indulge in (a) treat(s) – planned or not. What gets measured tends to get changed!
- **Cook at home.** You'll have more control over what you eat – what goes into your food, and how much of it you eat!   As a result your food log entries will be more accurate.
- **If improving athletic performance is one of your goals I highly encourage you to keep a detailed record of your workouts** including the weight used, your personal records (PRs), benchmarks, milestones, etc.

Be Mindful of the Process

Another thing that has worked well for me is to complete a **Weekly Progress Report** of sorts. Each week I take a few minutes to reflect on the previous seven days. Below is a list of the things I focus on. Feel free to use them as a guide:

o   *Describe how you are feeling (any significant thoughts, emotions, concerns, how you are feeling physically)*

o   *Describe what is happening in your body functions, energy levels, mood, outlook, etc.*

o   *Describe what is happening in your appearance.*

o   *Describe any changes in symptoms or conditions.*

o   *Describe your hunger between meals, satisfaction/satiety with meals. Note how you felt physically after eating.*

o   *Describe any changes in sleep (quality and/or duration).*

o   *Describe the best part of your week.*

o   *Talk about anything you struggled with during the week.*

o   *Note something you want/need to improve on in the coming week.*

Step 5 –
Describe Your Objective

The fact that you have stepped up to this challenge is, in itself, a success and proof of how strong you are. It's easy to say you want to improve or be better, but few people actually ever do anything about it. Why?? Because it's hard!!! Your desire to take this step shows that improving your health and well-being is a priority in your life. Congratulations!

During this process you will find and implement strategies that will work for you. You will figure out your problems and strengths and look at some options for finding a solution. Of course _you_ are the one who will be making decisions about lifestyle changes and, ultimately, implementing the lifestyle changes. I hope to be a source of expertise, support and inspiration.

Describe your current state of well-being.

Pull out your journal and complete the following sentences:

- *"I [your name] am fully committed to completing this program of transformation as it is presented to me." (Be sure to include today's date)*
- *"I am doing this because..."*
- *"My reward for following through with this process will be..."*

Describe your vision of yourself today.

- *How do you look?*

- *How do you feel?*
- *What aspects of your physical and mental well-being are disappointing to you?*

Describe your vision of yourself after completing this process.
- *What would it mean to look leaner, younger, better?*
- *What would it mean to feel younger, more fit, and full of energy?*
- *How would that feel?*
- *How will you know you are succeeding? What would that look like? (Be specific)*

What do you wish to achieve? (Please check all that apply).
- *improve athletic performance*
- *improve energy levels*
- *lose body fat*
- *reduce stress*
- *eliminate symptoms*
- *improve self-confidence*
- *improve mood*

Step 6 –

Assess Your Level of Motivation and Readiness to Change

Motivation is the underlying force for behavior change and there are varying levels of readiness to take action. In order to obtain a clearer picture of how *you* feel about change, two major components of readiness: importance and confidence – should also be assessed.

In a journal or notebook, please answer the following questions:

- *What are your S.M.A.R.T. goals?*
- *Why are your goals important to you? What motivates you?*
- *How long has this been an issue for you?*
- *What have you done in the past to try to achieve your goals? How many times have you tried?*
- *Why do you think you have failed so many times in the past?*
- *How committed are you to achieving your goals (Scale of 1-10)? If you answered less than 10, what would it take for you to be a 10?*
- *How ready are you to make some lifestyle changes in order to achieve your goals (Scale of 1-10)? If you answered less than 10, what would it take for you to be a 10?*

- *How important is it for you to make a change now (Scale of 1-10)? If you answered less than 10, what would it take for you to be a 10?*
- *How confident are you in your ability to achieve your goals (Scale of 1-10)? If you answered less than 10, what would it take for you to be a 10?*

More to think about...
- *What are your energy levels like during the day? (i.e. When do you have the most energy? When do you have the least energy?)*
- *Have you noticed a correlation between your food intake and your energy levels? Please describe.*
- *How many times have you been sick in the past year (cold, flu, etc.)?*
- *Are you currently taking any medication or supplements? If so, please list.*
- *Do you have any additional health concerns or medical issues that you have not mentioned? If so, please describe.*
- *Is there anything else you'd like to add?*

Check the phrase below that best describes where you are right now:
- ☐ Level 1 – Not motivated, not ready.
- ☐ Level 2 – Unsure, low confidence.
- ☐ Level 3 – Motivated, confident and ready!

Level 1 – Not motivated, not ready.

People at this level do not need *solutions*; they need to know they have a *problem*! In my experience, sometimes people are not aware of the benefits of behavior change or the risks and consequences of their present dietary behavior. They often know that improving their diet would probably be better for them. However they may not have given thought to how they would benefit personally or in which way they may feel better. Others have misconceptions about the type of dietary changes that are needed. I encourage you to keep reading.

Level 2 – Unsure, low confidence.

People in this category have indicated that diet change is possible but very little thought may have been given to exactly *what* is keeping them from making dietary changes. They know the problem exists but something is needed to push the decisional balance in favor of making a change. In my experience, people at this level know they need a solution but may not have all the facts regarding the benefits of changing. They may not really know what dietary changes would have to be made. Simple facts may be all that is needed to progress to a higher level of readiness to change.

I encourage you to explore your likes and dislikes about this issue by answering the following questions.

- *What do you like about your present diet?*
- *What do you dislike about your present diet?*
- *What do you think you would like about making a change to your present diet?*

- *What do you think you would dislike about making a change to your present diet?*

Now imagine the future. Imagine that you made all the changes necessary to achieve your health and wellness goals.

- *What is the first thing you notice that is different? What else is different?*
- *How do you feel?*
- *What does your spouse/significant other/family see you doing?*
- *Are any very small parts of this presently happening?*
- *How would you like your diet to be in the future?*

It also may help to explore past successes and identify abilities.

- *What strategies have you used in the past to overcome obstacles?*

For those at Level 1 or Level 2:

Ultimately these are all just **symptoms of much bigger problems** that come from:

1. Not having the *knowledge* of how to put a complete program together.
2. Not having a *workable plan of action* that integrates all components required for your success.
3. Not having the *support system* required to make the lifestyle changes necessary to not only achieve your goals, but also to maintain them for life.

MY HOPE IN WRITING THIS BOOK IS TO HELP YOU SOLVE THESE PROBLEMS.

Level 3 – Motivated, confident and ready!

People at this level have indicated that they are ready to make a lifestyle change. My hope is that this book serves as a resource for increasing awareness of possible alternatives for solving problems, clarifying goals, and tailoring behavior change strategies to achieve those goals. Please keep reading!

Whether you categorized yourself as Level 1, Level 2 or Level 3, you have options!!

In my experience, I have learned that different things work for different people. So I have come up with three different approaches depending on the client's level of motivation and readiness. All three approaches have been tried and tested by our clients (as well as yours truly) over the years. The end goal - a paleo lifestyle - is the same... but the path may look different for different people. You are free to choose what will work for you. I will outline each approach in _Step Twelve_.

Step 7 –

Get Rid of Your Scale

By following this plan as it is presented you can expect a gradual drop in body weight until normal healthy body weight is restored. For some people this may only take one or two months; for others, six months to a year; and for those with severe weight and health problems, a year or more. But the bottom line is *it will happen*. However, if weight loss is a goal, it's important that you understand that the focus during this process should be on making changes that *allow* weight loss to occur, not numbers on a scale. I urge you to not weigh yourself at any point. Your clothes don't lie. They either fit, or they don't. Use that as your guide.

I'll say it again (only louder). **IF WEIGHT LOSS IS A GOAL, IT'S IMPORTANT THAT YOU UNDERSTAND THAT THE FOCUS DURING THIS PROCESS SHOULD BE ON MAKING CHANGES THAT *ALLOW* WEIGHT LOSS TO OCCUR, *NOT* NUMBERS ON A SCALE.**

What the Scale Doesn't Measure

Here are just some of the things I experienced by following this plan that the scale can't measure:
Within days I noticed a dramatic improvement in my energy levels and sleep quality. I noticed my sinuses were clearer and my skin glowed. Within a week I actually started to notice a change in my body composition (with seemingly little effort). In less than two weeks I stopped craving the foods that at one point I couldn't imagine living

43

without (sugar, grains and starchy carbs). Over the next few weeks my bowel function normalized (Halleluiah!) and I no longer experienced the post-meal bloating and indigestion that I just attributed to overeating. My athletic performance improved – I got measurably faster and stronger. In less than 30 days (at the age of 35) I was looking, feeling and performing better than I ever had in my life!

Why I eat paleo

1) Eating this way does great things for my **mood, energy levels, body composition, complexion, quality of sleep, digestive health, bowel function, athletic performance**, etc. In short, I am quantifiably **leaner, healthier and stronger** when I eat paleo.

2) It helps me avoid hyperinsulinemia (http://en.wikipedia.org/wiki/Hyperinsulinemia) – also known as Syndrome X - which is responsible for hundreds of diet-induced illnesses and diseases – diabetes, high blood pressure, high cholesterol, metabolic syndrome, obesity...just to name a few.

3) Certain foods – grains, legumes, and dairy – cause **gut irritation and systemic inflammation**, which puts us at high risk for **autoimmunity** and a host of other problems

Nora T. Gedgaudas, author of <u>Primal Body - Primal Mind | Beyond the Paleo Diet forTotal Health and a Longer Life</u> sums it up beautifully:

"In the end, it's all a matter of what you prioritize. If health really matters to you, then the less you compromise it, the better. If superficial indulgence matters more...then I doubt you would be reading this. It's a choice we make. We need to make our choices more

consciously and thoughtfully—and less impulsively. Furthermore, the less you compromise your health, the easier it becomes not to compromise (you just don't get tempted after a while) AND the least likely you are to backslide and fall back into less healthy patterns of eating. —Like the Nike ad says: "Just Do It". Stick to your guns. Maintain your "health integrity". The ongoing and positively cumulative payoff will well exceed any superficial compromise to your impulsive desires. Your quality of life will not suffer in the absence of French fries, candy, potato chips, dessert or doughnuts. If you think it will, then you may need to take a look at what may be either addictions or a lack of healthy priorities."

Step 8 –
Differentiating Physical Hunger
vs. Emotional Hunger

When hunger or cravings occur during this process don't see it as an obstacle. Instead see it as an excellent learning opportunity! Differentiating between actual physical hunger and emotional hunger (cravings) is one of the most life-changing aspects of this program.

Examining, questioning, and redefining that thing we call hunger will free you from the traps you might be in around food.

- *Do you tend to eat too much food?*
- *Do you tend to eat the wrong kinds of food even though it negatively affects how you look, feel and perform?*
- *Do you lack the discipline to change your diet?*
- *Does food fill other roles in your life beyond nourishment and fuel causing you to eat without awareness?*

When the feeling of hunger creeps up, _before_ reacting (and eating) ask yourself:

"Is what I'm experiencing actual hunger? Or is it a craving?"

- *"Does it have anything to do with my body's actual need for calories and nutrients?*
    - *YES – It's hunger. Eat.*
    - *NO – It's a craving. It will pass.*

- *Or is it a need for something else: company, contact, forgiveness, acknowledgement, comfort, security....?"*
  - o *YES – It's a craving. It will pass.*
  - o *NO – It's hunger. Eat.*
- *"Would I eat a plate of steamed broccoli and baked chicken right now?"*
  - o *YES – It's hunger. Eat.*
  - o *NO – It's a craving. It will pass.*

Be mindful of exactly what you are feeling and where you are feeling it. Stay with the feeling. Describe it. Wait to see if it passes.. Drink a glass of water. (Often times thirst is confused for hunger)

As you pay attention to hunger start to notice:
- How often you habitually "feed" hunger the moment the feeling hits
- How often you reflexively reach for food out of habit when it is not actually needed for fuel.
- How uncomfortable the sensation is for you... *Is it so uncomfortable that you just want to get rid of it?*
- How often you eat because you are just bored and looking for stimulation or change

Once you are *aware* of a destructive habit you have the power to change it. Don't judge yourself or beat yourself up over it. Be grateful for the awareness and see it as an opportunity for growth!

As you learn to examine your "hunger" instead of immediately reacting to it you <u>will</u> develop the ability to take control over what you eat, when you eat, and how much of it you need to consume to feel your best.

Step 9 –
Behavior Change Strategies

If you want real results then knowing what to eat and what not to eat is essential. But it's just the tip of the iceberg and usually not enough to maintain a substantial food behavior change. As I've said before, the difference between success and failure for me meant a complete shift in my *thinking* and a change in my *behaviors*. Changing dietary behavior is a complicated process requiring numerous lifestyle adjustments. Let's be honest, change isn't easy and many times these adjustments can interfere with pleasurable activities. If substantial lasting results are a priority for you then keep reading!

Triggers occur normally throughout the day. For example, the feeling of hunger in our gut stimulates the desire to eat. We are particularly interested in cues that trigger *unconscious eating* or consumption of large quantities of certain types of food.

Some effective behavior change strategies can include:

- **Managing your triggers** – Identifying your triggers that produce detrimental behaviors (i.e. cause you to overeat) and then decreasing the occurrence by removing, avoiding or altering them. Identifying the triggers that produce positive behaviors and *increasing* the occurrence of those triggers.

- **Exchanging healthy responses for problem behaviors**

- **Providing rewards or punishment to regulate negative behaviors and strengthen positive behaviors.**

We will discuss each of these in detail in this chapter.

The sequence of events from *trigger to behavior to consequence* is referred to as a behavior chain.   Here are two examples:

- You come home from work very hungry. You walk into the kitchen to prepare dinner. There is a bag of your favorite potato chips on the counter (trigger). You tell yourself you will only eat a few and open the bag, leaving it on the counter as you prepare dinner. You end up eating the whole bag of chips (behavior). When dinner is ready, you pick at your food because you are not very hungry. You are frustrated because you know a bag of potato chips is not very nutritious and you are not getting enough lean protein, vegetables and healthy fat in your diet (negative consequence).

- You come home from work very hungry. There is a cup of berries and a slice of turkey in the fridge and workout clothes and sneakers prominently displayed on a chair in the kitchen (trigger). You eat the berries and sliced turkey, change your clothes, and go out for a jog (behavior). When you return, you are in good spirits, and you prepare dinner. You eat a healthy meal with lean protein, vegetables and healthy fat; you are content (positive consequence).

Now it's your turn. Take out your log and record one or more of your frequent behavior chains.

1. Identify the trigger

2. Specify the behavior

3. Describe the consequence (negative or positive)

Now, ask yourself:

- *Is this a behavior I would like to continue?*

- *If so, is there a way to encourage the occurrence of the trigger?*

- *If not, is there a way to alter the trigger or reduce the occurrence of it?*

Behavior Change Strategy: Managing Your Triggers

The first step in using this strategy is to identify your triggers. Triggers influence not only our desire to eat, but also what we eat, how much we eat, and how fast we eat. The triggers that we are particularly interested in are the ones that encourage *mindless* eating, poor food choices or consumption of large quantities of certain types of food. Our goal is to identify those triggers and remove them or at least reduce our exposure to them.

Sometimes triggers that stimulate a particular food response are obvious, but other times the triggers are not so obvious. For example, keeping an uncovered bowl of chocolate on your desk is an obvious trigger for anyone who enjoys chocolate. But did you know that such things as the placement of the food on the dinner table, the size of the plates you eat off of, the type of lighting in the room, and even the music that's playing during your meal can all be very powerful triggers causing you to eat more/faster?

I have found keeping a food log to be very helpful in identifying my triggers. As discussed in Step 4 – Keep a Log, some important details to record are: *detailed food intake and portion size, time of day, social setting (where you are and who you are with), your degree of hunger, your emotional state, and how a particular food makes you feel.*

Here are some rules I have set for myself based on triggers I have identified:

- **I designate one place in my home for eating all meals and snacks: the kitchen table.** I find that when I eat in many places of my home, each place becomes a trigger for eating – bed, office, living room, standing at the refrigerator with the door open.

- **Only eat when eating!** When I engage in activities, such as reading, texting, working on my laptop or driving a car while eating I tend to eat mindlessly. With fewer distractions, I can focus on the pleasures of eating and I'm more likely to notice (and stop eating) when I'm full.

- **I do not shop when hungry and I use a shopping list.** My degree of hunger can influence food purchases which encourages impulse buying. I typically eat before I go or, if I'm hungry when I arrive, I purchase something healthy from the cold food bar at Whole Foods and eat it before I begin shopping.

- **I serve foods in an attractive manner whenever possible**. For example I put a slice of lemon in a water glass or pour my sliced raw veggies into an attractive bowl.

- **I serve foods in the desired portion size and put away the rest**. For example, I count out the desired number of almonds into an attractive bowl and replace the bag in the cabinet. (Then I take the bowl to the kitchen table to eat).

- **During dinner, I leave serving dishes and pans in the kitchen** instead of on the table. Having them even a few steps away, as opposed to right in front of me, gives me a chance to think about whether or not I'm really hungry before I impulsively reach for seconds. However, **I do the opposite with salad and vegetables**. If I do decide I'm hungry for more food I'm more likely to reach for another serving of veggies if they are conveniently placed an arm's length away.

- **I bring snacks with me to the movies**. The movie theater is a big trigger for me. History has proven that it is nearly impossible for me to sit through a movie without eating *something*! So I bring beef jerky, kale chips, raw veggies (baby carrots, sugar snap peas and sliced bell pepper) and almond butter for dipping, or black olives to munch on. Otherwise the popcorn and pretzel bites are nearly impossible to resist!

- **I have learned to say "No, thank you" to offers of food.**

- **I prepare and portion my food into single serving containers.** I do this ahead of time as part of my Weekly Food Prep (a.k.a. my Sunday Ritual). That way when hunger strikes I can grab something quickly instead of having to fuss over a meal (and I can't use the "there's nothing to eat" excuse).

- **I plan and rehearse how to deal with temptations at an upcoming social event.** Parties and social gatherings can be particularly difficult for me. There is often an array of tempting foods, and if alcohol is consumed, my defenses decline.

- I have a snack ahead of time such as a hard-boiled egg, an apple and a small handful of almonds so I do not arrive hungry.
- I do much better when I drink water or club soda and decide (in advance) to have one or two alcoholic drinks, if any.
- I volunteer to bring a vegetable platter or other acceptable food for my needs. When I'm at the party I try to not stand near the food.

- **I slow down!!** If I suddenly find myself inhaling my meal I become more conscious of putting my utensils down between mouthfuls, chewing fully before swallowing, taking small bites, and swallowing each bite before adding any more food.

- **I set a goal to leave food on the plate** when I'm out at a restaurant. The helping is typically two or three times bigger than a regular serving size. I know that I can wrap half of it and enjoy leftovers the following day.

- **I stop eating when I'm no longer hungry** rather than when I'm full, knowing it takes about 20 minutes for my body and brain to signal satiation.

- **I store foods that should be avoided out of sight and in inconvenient places.** Whenever possible, I do not bring foods into the house that I am trying to avoid. But if it's there I at least store it in the back of the refrigerator, high up on a shelf, or in a cabinet that I don't regularly open.

- **I have found that family and friends can help or hinder my progress in sticking with my plan.** Here is a list of ways in which friends and family members can be supportive:
    - Help keep undesirable foods out of sight to avoid tempting triggers.
    - Purchase foods that I am trying to avoid in varieties that I do not like
    - Do not give foods to be avoided as gifts.
    - Offer praise and express appreciation for the accomplishment of difficult tasks.
    - Show patience for extra time needed to cook and prepare foods.
    - Avoid teasing or tempting me with foods that need to be avoided.
    - Avoid scolding, nagging and preaching. Although such behavior may be well intentioned, the overall effect is destructive.
    - Avoid using the words "strange" or "different" to describe my way of eating.

Behavior Change Strategy: Exchanging Healthy Responses for Problem Behaviors

If you simply stop a habit or pattern, there is likely to be a void unless a new behavior is substituted. For example, you may consume two cups of ice cream each night after dinner in front of the TV. The transition to changing that behavior will go more smoothly if an alternative behavior is planned, such as going for a walk, reading a book, or taking a bath.

Behavior Change Strategy: Providing Reward or Punishment to Regulate Negative Behaviors and Strengthen Positive Behaviors

In most cases, keeping a food log and managing my triggers has been adequate to develop and sustain desired behaviors; however when I need an added incentive to regulate and strengthen behavior, rewards can be sometimes be effective. For me, rewards (positive consequences) are more effective than punishment (negative consequences). Of course, to be effective, the reward would only come after the desired behavior, not before. Some rewards that work for me are:

- a new outfit or article of clothing
- a bubble bath
- taking a nap or "doing nothing"
- getting a massage
- getting a manicure or pedicure

Step 10 –
Go Paleo!

What Is Paleo?

Wikipedia provides this definition:

> *The Paleolithic diet, also popularly referred to as the caveman diet, Stone Age diet, and hunter-gatherer diet, is a nutritional plan based on the presumed ancient diet of wild plants and animals that various human species habitually consumed during the Paleolithic era – a period of about 2.5 million years duration that ended around 10,000 years ago with the development of agriculture. The diet consists mainly of grass-fed pasture-raised meats, fish, vegetables, fruit, roots, and nuts, and excludes grains, legumes, dairy products, salt, refined sugar, and processed oils.*

Base your diet on real, fresh, natural, nutrient-dense foods like meats, eggs and poultry, fish (rich in protein and good quality essential fats) a variety of vegetables (rich in antioxidants and cancer-fighting substances), healthy fats (like olive oil, avocados and coconut), and a small amount of fruit and nuts.

Avoid empty calories – high-calorie foods and drinks that offer little nutritional value. Eat foods that are **natural - not processed**. Avoid anything with grains (yes, even whole grains), legumes (that includes peanuts, hummus, edamame and any other products that contain soy), sugars and unhealthy fats.

Steer clear of anything that comes in a box or fancy packaging and is labeled "fat free," "low fat," "low carb", "heart healthy," etc.

Pay attention to where your food comes from. Whenever possible, buy meat that is grass-fed, local, organic and pastured, eggs that are organic and pastured, and produce that is locally and organically grown and in season.

Why I Eat Paleo?

Eating this way does great things for my mood, energy levels, body composition, complexion, quality of sleep, digestive health, bowel function, athletic performance, etc. In short, I am quantifiably leaner, healthier and stronger when I eat Paleo.

According to Dr. Michael Eades, author of The Protein Power Lifeplan (http://www.proteinpower.com/index.php), certain foods – **grains, legumes, and dairy** – cause gut irritation and systemic inflammation, which puts us at high risk for autoimmunity and a host of other problems. By adopting a paleo lifestyle, you'll maximize your insulin sensitivity, improve gut function, minimize autoimmune triggers, and optimize nutritional healing.

WHAT DOES 100% PALEO LOOK LIKE?

WHAT TO EAT...

[PROTEIN] Lean Meats, Fish, Poultry and Eggs

Lean beef (trimmed of visible fat)

Look for organic, grass-fed, locally farmed whenever possible

- Flank steak
- Top sirloin steak
- Extra-lean hamburger (no more than 7% fat, extra fat drained off)
- London Broil
- Chuck steak
- Lean veal
- Any other lean cut

Lean pork (trimmed of visible fat)

Look for organic, "pastured" whenever possible

- Pork loin
- Pork chops

Lean poultry (white meat, skin removed)

Look for organic, "pastured" whenever possible

- Chicken breast
- Turkey breast
- Game hen breasts

Eggs (Dr. Cordain suggests limiting consumption to six *whole* eggs per week)

Look for organic, "pastured," Omega-3 enriched whenever possible

- Chicken (go for the enriched omega 3 variety)
- Duck
- Goose

Fish

Look for wild caught

- o Bass
- o Bluefish
- o Cod
- o Drum
- o Eel
- o Flatfish
- o Grouper
- o Haddock
- o Halibut
- o Herring
- o Red Snapper
- o Salmon
- o Tuna
- o Any other commercially available fish

[CARBS] Produce

For ideal health, you should eat vegetables with every meal. Buy local, in season, organic produce whenever possible.

Fruits

ALL fruits except berries and melons (dried fruit, bananas, tropical fruit, etc.) should be consumed in moderation due to their high sugar content.

- o Blackberries*
- o Blueberries*
- o Raspberries*
- o Strawberries*
- o Apple*
- o Avocado
- o Blackberries*
- o Blueberries*
- o Raspberries*
- o Strawberries*
- o Cantaloupe
- o Cherries*
- o Grapefruit
- o Kiwi
- o Honeydew melon

Vegetables

(Limit starchy tubers like white potatoes, yams, and sweet potatoes to post-WOD meal only)

- Artichoke
- Asparagus
- Bell peppers
- Broccoli
- Brussels sprouts
- Cabbage
- Carrots*
- Celery*
- Cucumber

- Eggplant
- Green onions
- Lettuce*
- Mushrooms*
- Peppers (all kinds)*
- Pumpkin
- Spinach*
- Squash
- Tomato (actually a fruit)

*** = Produce that should be bought "organic"**

[FATS] Nuts and Seeds

Nuts and seeds are rich sources of monounsaturated fat. If you are trying to lose weight, you should eat no more than four ounces of nuts and seeds a day.

- Almonds
- Brazil nuts
- Hazelnuts
- Macadamias (best choice!)

- Pecans
- Pine nuts
- Sunflower seeds (and sunflower seed butter)
- Walnuts

[FATS] Oils, etc.

- Avocados (actually a fruit)
- Guacamole (check the label for non-Paleo ingredients)
- Coconut milk (from a can, NOT a carton)
- Coconut oil (great for cooking!)
- Coconut butter (usually in the oil aisle. Yummy!)
- Coconut flakes (no sulfites or added sugar)
- Olive oil (organic, cold pressed)

Beverages

- Water (bottled or filtered) – add a slice of lemon, lime, berries, or cucumber for flavor!
- Sparkling Water (bottled, unsweetened, and NO artificial sweeteners)
- Coffee (unsweetened, black or w/ a splash of coconut/almond milk)
- Tea (unsweetened, herbal)
- Kombucha

...For a more complete list, please read *The Paleo Diet* by Dr. Loren Cordain Ph. D.

WHAT TO AVOID...

Many authors and bloggers advocate what a strict 100% Paleo diet might look like and there are slight variations in each case. I believe the standards outlined below are a good place to start.

- Avoid ALL potential allergens:
  - **ALL cereal grains and gluten and products made from them** (even so-called healthy whole grains!) That means no wheat, oats, rice, corn, amaranth, rye, barley, cous cous, spelt, etc. For our purposes corn is also considered a grain.
  - **ALL beans and legumes.** This includes peanuts (Sorry, no peanut butter) and hummus! Cashew or almond butter (no sugar added) is just as good.
  - **ALL forms of soy.** This includes soybeans, edamame, tofu (meat substitute), soy sauce, and food additives (**Read your labels!** You'd be surprised by all the places you'll find soy)!
  - **ALL dairy products.** This includes milk, yogurt, cheeses, and butter solids. Not even cream in your coffee. Canned coconut milk (not from a carton) is a delicious alternative!
  - **If you have serious inflammation issues** like arthritis, you may want to consider avoiding nightshades as well.

  Check out *"How to Read a Label for a Wheat-Free, Peanut-Free, Soy-Free, Milk-Free Diet"* *(http://www.foodallergy.org/document.doc?id=133)*
- **Avoid ALL pro-inflammatory foods.** This includes starchy carbohydrates, grains, flours, and sugars as well as "trans fats" (partially hydrogenated oils).
- **Avoid ALL sugars.** This includes honey, agave, corn syrup, cane sugar, table sugar, etc. (**Read your labels!** You'll find forms of sugar hidden anywhere from tomato sauce and salad dressing to beef jerky and salsa)! **Check out** *"Other Names for Sugar That*

Appear On Labels" (http://www.fitsugar.com/Other-Names-Sugar-Appear-Labels-810571)

o **Avoid ALL processed foods.** This includes protein bars and shakes, as well as "Paleo" muffins, "Paleo" cookies, "Paleo" protein bars, "Paleo" pancakes, etc. The goal is to eat REAL food as close to its natural state as possible...NOT to "Paleo-ify" junk food!

o **Avoid ALL foods containing** preservatives, additives, chemicals and added sugars. (Look out for "hidden sources" such as sauces, condiments, salad dressings, etc. Read your labels).

o **Avoid ALL artificial sweeteners.** This includes saccharin (Sweet N Low), acesulfame K, cyclamate, aspartame (Equal), sucralose (Splenda)-*except the sweet herb stevia.*

o **Avoid ALL forms of alcohol.** This includes beer, wine, and distilled spirits.

o **Limit ALL sources of caffeine** to one or two single 6-ounce cup(s) of coffee (or one shot espresso) per day.

A Paleo Experiment

Now, I realize that eliminating grains, processed foods, legumes, dairy products, and sugar from your diet will be difficult for some people. It *will* take careful planning and preparation. It may mean packing a cooler... or making special requests when dining out. I challenge you to test it, experiment. Try it for yourself for 28 days (or more) and see the difference it makes in your life. You can do anything for one month. **Just think, you may be only 28 days away from feeling better than you ever have in your life!** Worst case scenario: You don't notice a significant change in your energy levels, your body composition and your athletic performance; you gave up some of your favorite foods for 28 days; you go back to what you were doing before. .

I know what you're probably thinking, "But I don't feel bad. I *really am* fine." That's what I thought too. You may have issues with certain foods and not even know it! The *ONLY* way to know for sure if you have an issue with certain foods is to *completely* remove them from your diet for at least 28 days. Then, if you choose, you can reintroduce them one-by-one and see if/how they affect you. The only way to figure out what an optimal diet for you looks like is to EXPERIMENT AND OBSERVE.

REMEMBER: IF YOU KEEP DOING WHAT YOU'VE BEEN DOING, AND KEEP EATING THE WAY YOU'VE BEEN EATING, YOU WILL CONTINUE TO GET THE SAME RESULTS

For Those "Considering" Paleo as a Way of Life

I eat Paleo because it works. So I tell people about it. If someone is interested and open to trying it for 28 days I am happy to share what I know and help in any way I can.

A common response I hear is: "I know I need to cut out sugar (etc.) but I can't live without _____ (oatmeal, whole grain bread, white potatoes, hummus, peanut butter, yogurt, etc.) ever again."

My reply: Let's be honest. It's not that you *can't* do it. You are *choosing* not to. Changing your eating habits takes effort and commitment. It may be difficult at first but isn't a lean, strong body, vibrant health, and a long life worth going without some of the foods you like for one month?

The fact that sugar is bad for your health (not to mention your waistline / the size of your butt) doesn't come as a surprise to most people and a person with any common sense knows it should be avoided. But some people are very resistant to even the idea of giving up (so called healthy) grains, legumes, and dairy products. I know I was at first. I realize that food is a very emotional thing for most people and I have had enough experience to know that people will not change until *they* are motivated to change. I believe wholeheartedly – without exception – that *everyone* can benefit from a paleo way of eating. But I don't want you to just take *my* word for it!

I think it's an accurate assumption that you are reading this book because what you have been doing isn't working for you and you need help. If you find yourself resistant to even trying paleo for 28 days I challenge you to ask yourself the following questions:

o   *Is the way you are eating now working miracles for you? Is this way of eating enabling you to lose weight (and/or keep it off) effortlessly?*

o   *Why do you believe that the way you are eating is better? Is it just because it has been drilled into your head by food marketers, the media, and/or so called experts?*

o   *Has your current way of eating made you quantifiably healthier, leaner, and stronger?*

o   *Why are you so resistant to changing your eating habits and at least trying Paleo for 28 days? Is it because you are lazy or afraid? (Be honest) Or could it be that you are so (physically and/or emotionally) addicted to certain foods that you just can't bear to live without them – not even for 28 days?*

A Paleo "Template"

In his **9 Steps to Perfect Health** series
(http://chriskresser.com/perfecthealth) Chris Kresser attempts to
define the general dietary guidelines that constitute what he calls a
"Paleo Template."

Step 1 – Don't Eat Toxins

- Cereal grains (especially refined flour)
- Omega-6 industrial seed oils (corn, cottonseed, safflower, soybean, etc.)
- Sugar (especially high-fructose corn syrup)
- Processed soy (soy milk, soy protein, soy flour, etc.)

Step 2 – Nourish Your Body

- Get away from thinking of food as macronutrients ("low-fat" or "low-carb" or "high-protein") and start thinking of food as a means of nourishment and fuel. *"This means we classify foods not based on their macronutrient ratios but on their ability to provide the energy and nutrition the body needs to function optimally."*

Step 3 – Eat Real Food

- Whole, unprocessed and unrefined
- Pasture-raised (i.e. grass-fed) and wild
- Local, seasonal and organic

You can check out all **9 Steps to Perfect Health** *at
(http://chriskresser.com/perfecthealth)*

I personally agree with the idea of a Paleo "template" for two reasons:

1. Finally, we can get rid of the word "diet"
2. It allows for some flexibility and experimenting while staying within certain guidelines.

...BUT (and there is a but) I wholeheartedly believe that *everyone* should go through a period of elimination and reintroduction – completely removing grains, dairy, and legumes for no less than 28 days BEFORE transitioning to a Paleo "template." The introduction of a template is not permission to pick and choose, following the advice that you like and ignoring the rest without really knowing whether a certain food is having a negative impact on your health.

I've done the strict 28-40 days of paleo several times and have found that I don't respond well to gluten, grains and legumes. But I can tolerate *small amounts* of (some) dairy products, such as grass-fed heavy cream, raw milk cheese. But I never would have discovered my sensitivity without a period of elimination and reintroduction, since I had been eating them for years and I felt "fine."

Even though I am not one hundred percent paleo one hundred percent of the time (I am human, after all), I am still relatively strict (I'll take you through a typical day for me in Step Thirteen). I eat this way to optimize my health. And as long as I continue to look, feel and perform the way I like, I will continue to do so.

For more information on Paleolithic nutrition, I recommend reading one (or all) of the great books listed in the Links and Resources section in the back of this book.

Primal Body – Primal Mind | Beyond the Paleo Diet for Total Health and a Longer Life , It Starts With Food, The Protein Power Lifeplan, The Paleo Diet (revised), The Paleo Solution, The Primal Blueprint.

I also get a lot of information from Nora T. Gedgaudas (http://www.primalbody-primalmind.com/) , Drs. Michael and Mary Dan Eades (http://proteinpower.com/) , Dr. Loren Cordain (http://thepaleodiet.com/) , Robb Wolf(http://robbwolf.com/) , Chris Kresser (http://chriskresser.com/) , and Mark Sisson (http://www.marksdailyapple.com/)

Step 11 –
Carb-ivore No More!

For years we were told by so called experts that if we just ate less fat and more carbohydrates we would be improving our diets and we would all get skinnier! I bought into it just like most other Americans. The sad truth is it took over a decade for me to accept that the low-fat / high-carb thing wasn't working for me. I was completely frustrated and didn't know what to try next. But there were three things I knew for sure:

1. My diet was loaded with empty calories – low-fat processed foods with lots of added sugar but few (or no) nutrients.
2. I struggled with weight gain, despite my efforts eat fewer calories and exercise more.
3. I was addicted to carbohydrates. I suffered from uncontrollable cravings and once I started eating a high carbohydrate food I found it very difficult to stop.

In the late 1990s and early 2000s came the "low-carb craze" when low carbohydrate diets like The Atkins Diet and other diets with similar principles became the most popular diets in the country. I was intrigued… Okay, I was desperate. So I jumped on the low-carb bandwagon. I was allowed unlimited consumption of salty fatty meats and cheeses, but all foods containing carbohydrates, including fruits were off limits. To my surprise and delight, I actually started getting leaner. But I couldn't shake the belief that I was achieving short-term weight loss at the expense of long-term health. And none of it was sustainable as a way of life. I still found myself on a diet then off a diet then back on a diet... and every Monday was day one.

Then I heard about Dr. Barry Sears' 'Zone Diet' (http://zonediet.com/). The Zone is about keeping hormonal responses (in particular, the hormone insulin) generated by the food you eat within a zone: not too high (which would prevent you from accessing stored body fat for energy), not too low (which would cause your cells to starve to death). According to Dr. Sears, *every* meal and snack should have a 30%-40%-30% ratio of protein, carbohydrate and fat. This ideal ratio would be just enough protein, carbohydrates and fat to support exercise and daily activities, but not body fat. Fortunately, as you'll see, that isn't as complicated as it sounds. Keep reading for some tips on building meals and snacks. (For more information read The Zone by Barry Sears, Ph.D.)

According to Dr. Barry Sears who developed the Zone Diet, food should be understood as a drug that stimulates a powerful hormonal response. It goes a little something like this:

> When you eat, blood sugar (glucose) rises. This rise in blood sugar signals the release of the hormone insulin. Insulin's job is to drive down blood sugar levels (too much glucose is toxic for the body). Insulin does its job by acting as a key to unlock insulin receptors on the surfaces of the cells. These receptors pump the glucose out of the blood and drive it into muscle, liver, and fat cells where it can be burned for energy or stored as fuel for later use. Here's the hitch: Eating more carbohydrates results in more insulin production. The storage capacity of muscle and liver cells is pretty

low. When your muscle and liver cells have reached their maximum storage capacity, any remaining glucose is converted into fat and sent to the fat cells for storage. One of insulin's jobs as the primary nutrient-storage hormone is to transport fat into the fat cells. When we eat too much carbohydrate we are basically sending a message to the body to store fat.

The counter-hormone to insulin is glucagon. Decreased blood sugar – or hunger – signals the release of glucagon. Glucagon's job is to normalize or restore blood sugar and energy levels by releasing stored glucose (glycogen) while allowing you better access to your stored body fat for energy (That's a good thing). Insulin and glucagon work together to manage energy and body fat levels. When insulin levels are high, the release of glucagon is inhibited and metabolism is impaired. In other words, not only do increased insulin levels tell the body to store carbohydrate as fat, they tell it not to release any stored body fat for energy.

In order to get the stored fat out of the fat cells and burn it for energy – that is, to reduce body fat – insulin levels must drop. If insulin levels are low enough, fat storage comes to a halt. (Remember, fat can't get into the fat cells without the help of insulin). In order for insulin levels to drop, your system must become more responsive to its effects (insulin sensitivity). If the high-glucose/insulin pattern continues (i.e. you continue eating a high-carb diet) the result is weight gain and insulin resistance. Therefore, it's crucial to keep insulin levels low by controlling your carbohydrate intake. (For more information read *The Protein*

Power Lifeplan by Michael R. Eades, M.D. and Mary Dan Eades, M.D.)

The key is learning how to control hormonal responses through diet. According to Dr. Sears, the critical hormonal balance of insulin and glucagon depends on two things:

1. The size of the meal you eat – Excess calories stimulate the secretion of insulin.
2. The ratio of protein to carbohydrate in each meal.

Step 12 –

Choose an Approach

I have learned over the years that different things work for different people. So I have come up with three different approaches for you to choose from depending on your level of commitment and readiness.

- Level One – 100% Paleo
- Level Two – The Open Meal Approach
- Level Three – The One-Meal-at-a-Time Approach

While the general principle is the same – that the progressive elimination of certain foods or groups of foods that are potential allergens (such as grains, processed foods, legumes, dairy products, and sugar) will lower insulin and ultimately lead to health benefits – the level of restriction varies.

How should I choose which level to start at?

Do I think everyone should permanently eliminate grains, processed foods, legumes, dairy products and sugar from their diet? Not necessarily. Not everyone has issues with or suffers sensitivities to these foods. You may be thinking, "I know I don't have issues with these foods. I eat them every day and I'm fine." Not so fast! Remember, the only way to truly know if certain foods are having a negative effect is to cut them out completely for 28 days (or more)...then *slowly* reintroduce those foods one by one (if you choose) and notice the impact they have on how you look, feel and perform. Elimination diets can be a very effective means of determining the potential for food sensitivity. But 100 percent adherence is required to make a clear determination. For that reason, I believe everyone should *start* at Level One, figure out for themselves what foods are having a negative effect, and then transition to a variation of Level 2 based on what they discover.

Level Two (The Open Meal Approach) and Level Three (The One-Meal-at-a-Time Approach) will allow you to "ease" into Paleo over a three-week period but my experience has overwhelmingly shown that it is much more effective (and far less painful) to simply eliminate non-paleo foods and get your body used to using fat, rather than sugar, as a primary source of fuel. However, if you are a beginner (or if you described yourself as "unsure, low confidence" in Step Six) you may want to adhere to Level Two or Level Three before you move to Level One.

All three plans have been tried and tested by our clients (*and* yours truly) over the years. It's not a one-size-fits-all approach. What works for one person may not work for another. I encourage you to experiment and figure out what works for you. The end goal – a sustainable plan, real results, lasting change, and a paleo lifestyle – is the same... but the path may look different for different people.

LEVEL ONE | 100% PALEO

*This is the strictest regimen, one that closely mimics the diet our ancient hunter-gatherer ancestors thrived on and therefore bestows the **maximum health and fitness rewards**. I believe that EVERYONE* *should start here. The period of time you spend at this level will vary depending on your weight-loss goals and your current state of health. It may take only a few weeks to alter blood sugar, cholesterol, triglycerides, or blood pressure, for example, but it could take several months to lose a substantial amount of weight. Once you have completed this stage you will complete seven days of reintroduction (I'll talk about this in Step Fifteen – Reintroduction). After completing your reintroduction you may choose to move to Level Two for maintenance (except for those with chronic disease, who may do better with long-term adherence to strict paleo). You can always return to Level One in the future anytime you feel you have gotten off track.*

- 100% paleo for 28 days to several months (depending on your weight-loss goals and your current state of health).

Have I adopted the stringent approach described above? Yes, I have. Do I believe it's the optimal nutritional strategy for me to reap the maximum degree of wellness possible? Yes, I do. Do I maintain this degree of restriction at all times? No, I don't. In September 2012 we had a "Paleo Experiment" at our gym where clients were challenged to go 100% paleo for 31 days. I participated in the 31-day challenge as well. For the duration of the challenge I kept a detailed log of my experience and I published my log entries on my blog. My log included not only what and how much I ate but also a daily summary of my sleep, energy and motivation levels, any significant thoughts, emotions or insights regarding my nutrition... and anything else that came to mind. Keeping a food log – and publishing it to my blog - helped keep me focused and accountable.

Check it out!

http://www.transformcrossfit.com/traceys_blog/2012/09/index.html

LEVEL TWO | THE OPEN MEAL APPROACH

This is a middle-of-the road plan for those people who will accept slightly more restriction for better health but may not be ready for Level One (If you described yourself as "unsure, low confidence" in Step Six). Level Two is also a good transition/maintenance plan after completing 28+ days of 100% paleo (It is, in fact, the way I eat most of the time).

- Week One - Focus on going strict paleo allowing for no more than THREE "open" meals (off-plan treats) for the first seven days.
- Week Two - Focus on going strict paleo allowing for no more than TWO "open" meals for the next seven days.
- Week Three - Focus on going strict paleo allowing for no more than ONE "open" meal for the next seven days.

LEVEL THREE | THE ONE-MEAL-AT-A-TIME APPROACH ("Beginner")

This plan is the least restrictive of all, at least in the beginning. if you are a beginner (or if you described yourself as "unsure, low confidence" in Step Six) you may want to start here before you move to Level One or Level Two.

- Week One - Focus on having a 100% paleo breakfast every day for seven consecutive days.

- Week Two - Focus on having a 100% paleo breakfast <u>and</u> lunch every day for seven consecutive days.
- Week Three - Focus on having a 100% paleo breakfast, lunch, <u>and</u> dinner every day for seven consecutive days.

Step 13 –
Preparation

We've all heard the saying, "If you fail to plan you plan to fail." That statement is true whether you are talking about your business, your finances, or *your nutrition*. Eating right doesn't just happen by chance. It takes effort and commitment. If it were easy the obesity rate wouldn't be what it is today! As hard as we try, none of us can eat a perfect diet 100 percent of the time. But with just a little bit of careful planning and preparation you can improve the way you eat 95 percent of the time. If you can do that, then the occasional splurge (the other 5 percent) won't completely sabotage your efforts.

Action Plan

1. Preparation: Every week
2. Elimination (Level One | 100% Paleo): 28 days to several months depending on your weight-loss goals and your current state of health
3. Reintroduction: Seven days
4. Maintenance (Level Two | Open Meal Approach): Ongoing…

Schedule It In

I will go into each item in detail but here is a sample schedule. I strongly encourage you to pull out your calendar and schedule these things in. Treat them just as you would any other appointment.

Before you begin

- o Schedule Kitchen Clean Out (If you are not comfortable with throwing food away why not donate it!)

Every week

- o Plan meals and snacks for each day of the week.
- o Schedule Grocery Shopping trip to Whole Foods, health food store, farmer's market and/or supermarket (as long as they have a good organic selection)
- o Schedule Weekly Food Prep – Cook, chop, prep and portion out foods (I'll describe my Weekly Food Prep later in this chapter)
- o Complete a Weekly Progress Report (You can find a sample in *Step Four – Keep a Log*)

Every day

- o Complete your food log
- o Plan and prepare meals and snacks for the following day

Build a Meal... Easy as 1, 2, 3!

Having a specific template to structure each meal around will help you stay mindful. I have been following a modified version of Dr. Barry Sears' Zone Diet off and on since 2009 (See Step Eleven – Carbivore No More). I like having an accurate and precise prescription to go on because it allows me to figure out my baseline and then assess what is and isn't working. I initially committed to strict adherence to the Zone parameters in combination with the paleo way of eating and I benefited greatly. That is, I observed measurable improvements in athletic performance and body composition. I believe the 30%-40%-30 ratio is a good place to start. But after several years of trial and error and self-experimentation I have come up with a modified version of the Zone Diet that works very well for me. I discovered that when I increase the amount of fat that I add to my meals by up to two times I am able to sustain my energy levels and athletic performance while still maintaining a level of leanness that I am happy with. In a typical day (based on my weight, height, activity level and body composition) I eat approximately 75-80 grams of protein, 100 grams or less of carbohydrate, and around 35-50 grams of fat. I typically eat three meals and two snacks per day and the breakdown looks a little something like this:

1 Meal =

- 21 grams of protein
- 27 grams (or less) of low-glycemic carbohydrates
- 9-14 grams of fat

1 Snack =

- 7 grams of protein
- 9 grams (or less) of low-glycemic carbohydrates
- 3-5 grams of fat

**Please note that the above amounts are what I have found to work for me. Individual nutritional needs vary based on a person's weight, height, activity level and body composition.

Since strict adherence to the Zone Diet requires weighing and measuring everything you eat I'm not suggesting that the diet is sustainable for everyone. However, I highly encourage you to pull out your food scales and measuring cups, and weigh and measure portions for at least one week when you are at home. I think you will find that even after just one week you will develop the ability to "eyeball" portions when you don't have scales and measuring cups available. (I have found that when I "guesstimate" I tend to underestimate my portion sizes, especially when it comes to proteins and fats. So even after all this time I still weigh and measure).

As I talked about in *Step Four – Keeping a Food Log*, most people, it seems, are not very good at estimating how many calories they have eaten at a given meal or over the course of a typical day. It seems that most people are just as bad at estimating portion sizes and tend to underestimate how much they are actually eating. We consider a serving to be pretty much whatever we eat in one sitting. What you estimated to be a single (four-ounce) serving of chicken breast was probably actually six or seven ounces (up to two servings). A single serving of granola is ¼ cup. That "small bowl" of granola you had for breakfast was likely triple an actual serving size. If it was labeled "low-fat" you probably ate even more because you told yourself it was "healthy." That handful of almonds that you estimated to be a single serving (one-quarter cup), in reality was probably twice that. If you were eating from a big, multi-serving bag you probably considered whatever amount you ate to be "one serving." **Even if it's something you believe is healthy, too much of a good thing is still too much and can result in weight gain.**

To achieve blood glucose control, <u>every</u> meal *and* snack should contain some protein, carbohydrates and fat. Here is a good template to follow when building a meal or snack:

1. Start with protein.

2. Add in your carbs – Emphasize vegetables. Fruit should be more of a condiment or dessert... and it's completely optional.

3. Add in some healthy fat.

Step 1 - Start with PROTEIN

Protein should be the first thing you should consider when putting together a meal or snack. Begin by dividing your plate into three equal parts. On one-third of your plate, add one serving of lean protein that is no bigger or thicker than the palm of your hand. That's about three ounces for women and four ounces for men. Portion sizes for snacks will be about one-third or one-half that amount. Protein should be cooked simply, without too much added fat - broiling, baking, roasting, sautéing, or browning, then pouring off excess liquid fat, or stir frying over high heat with a little coconut oil.

Step 2a – Add in your vegetables (CARBS)

Fill the remaining two-thirds of your plate with non-starchy vegetables. For ideal health I try to eat vegetables with every meal. I like to aim for at least two different types of vegetables and two different colors (at least one full serving of each) at each meal/snack to add variety and avoid boredom. Emphasize a variety of vegetables throughout the day – especially leafy greens – and eat A LOT of them! Fruit should be enjoyed as a condiment or dessert. Buy local, in season, organic produce whenever possible.

Step 2b (optional) – Add in your fruit (CARBS) -

If your primary goal is fat loss you may want to keep your fruit intake down to one or two servings per day or eliminate it altogether for a while. To those who fall into that category, Robb Wolf (http://robbwolf.com/), author of The Paleo Solution suggests making most of your meals protein, vegetables and fat. There is no nutrient in fruit that is not available in vegetables and most fruits tend to be higher in carbohydrates (sugar). If you are already lean and/or you are an athlete, you may be able to get away with more fruit (and starchy tubers like yams and sweet potatoes).

Serving size will vary depending on the fruit. The serving size for berries is typically between ½ and one cup. One cup is roughly the size of an average woman's fist or a baseball. One-half cup of berries fits in the palm of your hand with your hand open. Many fruits carry relatively high glycemic values and low antioxidant values and should be enjoyed in moderation if at all and careful attention should be paid to portion size. These include bananas, all dried fruits, oranges, tangerines, grapes, plums, melons, mangoes, papayas, pineapples, and pomegranates. In general it's best to avoid fruit juices and eat the whole fruit instead. However, fruit juice is great to use as a sweetener in homemade salad dressings and condiments.

Step 3 – Add in your FATS

Add a dash of heart healthy fat such as avocado, olive oil, guacamole, slivered almonds or walnuts. One ounce of nuts is roughly the size of a *small* closed handful. One ounce of nut butter is about the size of your thumb. Two tablespoons of nut butter is about the size of a golf ball. One teaspoon of oil is roughly the size of the *tip* of your thumb or the size of one die.

Meal and Snack Ideas (PRO + CARBS + FAT)

Try to keep your meals small. Every meal and snack should contain some protein, carbohydrates and fat. For ideal heath, you should eat a serving of lean protein and low-glycemic, non-starchy vegetables with every meal, along with moderate amounts of fruit, nuts, avocados, seeds, and healthful oils.

Breakfast

- Scrambled, poached, or hardboiled Omega 3 enriched eggs (PROTEIN) + a small handful of fresh berries (CARBS) + avocado slices (FAT)
- Ground chicken sausage (PROTEIN) browned and sautéed in coconut oil (FAT) served over mashed cauliflower (total comfort food!)
- A frittata loaded with veggies (PROTEIN + CARBS) is a great option since it can be made ahead of time and eaten later, either hot or cold. Add a small handful of olives (FAT).
- Baked "ham and egg cups" (PROTEIN) + organic strawberries (CARBS) + sunflower seed butter (FAT)
- An omelet (PROTEIN) filled with veggies (CARBS) – hold the cheese and skip the toast!
- Smoked salmon (PROTEIN) + raw bell pepper slices (CARBS) + macadamia nuts (FAT)

- Grass-fed sirloin leftover from last night's dinner (PROTEIN) + sautéed apples and pecans (CARBS + FAT)

Lunch / Dinner Ideas

- Lean meat, fish or poultry (PROTEIN) + A large green salad (CARBS) + olive oil (FAT) and lemon juice
- Homemade chicken salad (PROTEIN + FAT) wrapped in butter lettuce (You'll never miss bread!)
- Uncured, nitrate-free lunch meat (PROTEIN) piled on top of salad greens (CARBS) + olive oil (FAT) and vinegar.
- Ground beef and/or chicken (PROTEIN) browned and sautéed in coconut oil (FAT) with a serving or two of grilled vegetables (CARBS).
- Beef and/or chicken Fra Diavolo (PROTEIN + CARBS) over steamed julienned zucchini and yellow squash (You'll never miss spaghetti!)
- Pork sirloin (PROTEIN) + roasted Brussels sprouts with walnuts (CARBS + FAT) + mashed cauliflower
- Grass-fed sirloin (PROTEIN) + cauliflower "rice" (CARBS) + grilled asparagus (CARBS) drizzled in olive oil (FAT)
- Grass-fed beef burger (PROTEIN) topped with guacamole (FAT) + homemade baked sweet potato fries (CARBS)
- Homemade tuna salad (PROTEIN + FAT) stuffed into one half of a red bell pepper (CARBS) or wrapped in butter lettuce.
- Leftovers from last night's dinner are also a convenient option.

- Almond stuffed dates wrapped in bacon (CARBS + FAT) + beef jerky (PROTEIN) – Look for natural products with a few seasonings listed, make your own.
- Paleo Kits (http://www.stevespaleogoods.com/Default.asp)
- Hard-boiled egg (PROTEIN) + baby carrots and celery sticks (CARBS) + almond butter (FAT)
- Sliced turkey breast (PROTEIN) + sliced bell peppers sprinkled with sea salt (CARBS) + guacamole (FAT).
- Canned or bagged tuna or sardines (PROTEIN) + carrots (CARBS) + olives (FAT)

One way to make this diet work for you is to always have paleo-friendly food available. A few helpful tips:

- Double or triple the size of your evening meal and bring the leftovers for lunch
- Cook two or more main dishes at night, use one and refrigerate the other for later in the week.
- Purchase precut washed salad vegetables and lettuces

Instead of This…Eat This.

A meal or recipe does not need to include wheat, grains, dairy, legumes, sugar or soy to be delicious. With a little creativity you can turn just about meal into a paleo-friendly meal. I always get the question "So what do I eat instead of _____?" Here are a few easy swaps I have learned to help turn your go-to "pre-paleo" meals into paleo-licous meals

- *Instead of sausage and grits*: ground chicken sausage over mashed cauliflower.
- *Instead of traditional pancakes with butter and syrup:* paleo pumpkin pancakes topped with coconut butter or almond butter.
- **Instead of eggs, toast with butter and home fries**: a vegetable omelet and a slice of coconut Paleo Bread (http://www.julianbakery.com/) with coconut butter or ghee.
- *Instead of popcorn at the movies*: a Paleo Kit (http://www.stevespaleogoods.com/Default.asp) or raw vegetables dipped in almond butter.
- *Instead of oatmeal or cereal*: primal hot cereal.
- *Instead of a peanut butter and jelly sandwich on whole grain bread*: sunflower seed butter and 100% fruit spread on Paleo Bread (http://www.julianbakery.com/).
- *Instead of apple pie*: sautéed apples and pecans.
- *Instead of white or whole grain tortillas or bread*: coconut wraps (http://www.improveat.com/) or Paleo Bread (http://www.julianbakery.com/).
- *Instead of spaghetti/pasta with meatballs*: julienne zucchini "spaghetti" or spaghetti squash topped with beef Fra Diavolo.
- *Instead of milk or cream*: unsweetened almond milk, hemp milk or canned coconut milk.
- *Instead of alcohol, wine or beer*: club soda with lime or Kombucha.
- *Instead of soy sauce*: coconut aminos.

- *Instead of peanut butter*: sunflower seed butter, almond butter, or coconut butter.

- *Instead of mashed (white) potatoes*: homemade mashed sweet potatoes.

- *Instead of French fries*: homemade baked sweet potato fries.

- *Instead of potato chips*: kale chips, beef jerky or plantain chips (no added sugar).

- *Instead of cappuccinos or lattes*: Americanos.

- *Instead of store bought mayo and salad dressing*: make your own (Mashed avocado is also a great substitute for mayo).

- *Instead of butter:* coconut oil or ghee (clarified butter).

Kitchen Clean-Out

Today's the day! Clean out your cabinets, refrigerator, pantry and anywhere else you store food and get rid of *any and all* non-Paleo items *(Hint: If it's been sitting on a shelf for any amount of time you can bet it's not paleo-friendly).* Strong willpower and good intentions typically don't cut it - If it's there you'll be way too tempted to eat it (I know I would be)!   Don't wait another minute. No excuses. (If you're "keeping it for the kids or spouse" they don't need it any more than you do!) Get up, grab a trash bag and do it right now! If you don't like the idea of throwing food away DONATE IT!! You'll be glad you did.

Weekly Meal Plan

It helps me to plan, in advance whenever possible, what my meals will look like each day of the week. Here is a sample of a typical day for me:

Meal 1 – (This meal is relatively small since it's typically very early in the morning. I just need a little something about an hour after I wake up but I'm not hungry enough for a full meal)

1 c coffee

1 turkey egg cup

1 cup mashed cauliflower or Brussels sprouts (or some other vegetable)

1 tsp almond butter

Meal 2 – (This is usually my post-workout meal)

3 oz. chicken breast

½ apple (chopped and sautéed in coconut oil and cinnamon)

¼ c sweet potato (baked)

3 tsp almond butter

Meal 3 –

3 oz. ground turkey or chicken breast over

1 ½ c zucchini "spaghetti" (steamed) and ½ c spicy tomato sauce

9 olives

¼ avocado

Meal 4 – (varies)

3 oz. lean protein (pork sirloin, chicken sausage, 85% lean grass-fed beef)

large "layered" salad (i.e. arugula, spring mix, spinach, chopped bell peppers, tomatoes, cucumber, sliced strawberries, avocado, nuts, homemade dressing)

Grocery Shopping (based on meal plan for the week)

Once you have planned your meals and snacks for the week and removed all off-plan items from your kitchen, it's time to stock up on the wide selection of food you will be eating! Below is a sample of my grocery list (enough for seven days for two people). If you are shopping for more than two people, obviously you'll need to purchase more food. This list includes the food I'll need for breakfast, lunch, and snacks - the foods I pack and carry with me - and dinner.

PROTEIN

- ☐ 1 ½ - 2 lbs. organic boneless skinless chicken breast
- ☐ 1 lb. grass-fed ground beef
- ☐ 1 ½ - 2 lbs. ground chicken or turkey breast
- ☐ 1 ½ - 2 lbs. ground chicken sausage
- ☐ 1 lb. pork sirloin
- ☐ 2-3 packages Brat Hans Organic Chicken Sausage
- ☐ 3 dozen organic cage-free pastured eggs
- ☐ 1 family sized package of Applegate Organics Organic Roasted Turkey Breast

PRODUCE (depending on what is in season)

- ☐ 1-2 containers organic berries
- ☐ 4 organic apples
- ☐ 6 bell peppers (red, orange and yellow)
- ☐ 1 bag baby carrots
- ☐ 1 lb. sugar snap peas
- ☐ 2 cucumbers
- ☐ 1 red onion
- ☐ 1 white onion

- [ ] 2-3 sweet potatoes
- [ ] 2 lbs. Brussels sprouts
- [ ] 1 lb. asparagus spears
- [ ] 1 – 11 oz. container organic spring mix or arugula
- [ ] 1 – 11 oz. container organic baby spinach
- [ ] 2 jars Newman's Own Fra Diavolo Sauce
- [ ] 1 or 2 10-oz. bags frozen butternut squash
- [ ] 1 or 2 heads organic cauliflower
- [ ] 1-2 bags frozen broccoli florets
- [ ] 1 jar minced garlic

FAT

- [ ] extra virgin olive oil
- [ ] coconut oil spray
- [ ] 1 jar raw organic coconut butter
- [ ] 1-2 lbs. nuts (usually walnuts, almonds and/or macadamias)
- [ ] 1 jar coconut oil
- [ ] 1 jar almond butter
- [ ] 2-4 organic avocadoes
- [ ] 2 cans olives

MISCELLANEOUS

- [ ] balsamic vinegar
- [ ] lemon juice
- [ ] coconut aminos
- [ ] Paleo Bread (grain-free, coconut or almond)
- [ ] coffee

Weekly Food Prep...For Time (of course!)

I'd like to invite you into my "virtual kitchen." I'm going to take you through my Sunday Ritual of preparing, cooking and portioning my meals for the week. I am a small business owner. I have a very hectic schedule and I work up to 60 hours some weeks. Even when I am home, oftentimes I am still working. Early mornings, late evenings, busy days... Sound familiar? But that doesn't keep me from eating a healthy paleo + zone diet. And all it takes is one hour of cooking and preparation per week. In just one hour I can prepare all my meals to last me from Monday to Friday. My weekly food prep will vary depending on my tastes and preferences at the time but here is a sample:

Let's get started!! 3...2...1...GO!

Start time: 2:14pm

- Preheat oven to 350 degrees
- Prepare **Turkey Egg Cups** (ingredients: 9-12 organic pastured eggs, organic nitrate-free turkey (or ham), coconut spray oil for muffin pan).
    - Spray muffin pan with coconut oil spray.
    - Line each cup with one slice of organic, nitrate-free turkey.
    - Carefully crack one organic pastured egg into each cup.
    - Season with salt, pepper and basil to taste and bake at 350 degrees for around 22 minutes.

- While the egg cups are baking, begin the **Chicken/Turkey Fra Diavolo** (Ingredients: 1 lb. ground chicken sausage, 1 lb. ground chicken breast, 1 jar Newman's Own Fra Diavolo spicy tomato sauce, coconut oil).
    - Melt about 1 tablespoon of coconut oil in saucepan over medium heat.
    - Add ground meat (I like a mixture of organic chicken sausage and chicken breast) and cook until all pink is gone.
    - Add the tomato sauce, cover and simmer for several minutes. Remove from heat and allow to cool.
- For **Baked Chicken Breast** place 1 lb. raw organic chicken breast to an 8x8 pan and cover with aluminum foil.
- Prepare **Roasted Brussels Sprouts with Walnuts** (Ingredients: 2 lbs. Brussels sprouts, walnuts, coconut oil spray)
    - Slice Brussels sprouts in half and add to a pan sprayed with coconut oil spray
    - Add walnuts (halves and pieces).
    - Add salt and pepper to taste.
- While the egg cups are cooking, continue prepping the rest of the **vegetables and fruit** (sliced bell peppers and cucumbers, julienned zucchini, etc.)...I like to fill one half bell pepper with the Ground Meat Fra Diavolo mixture, or just sprinkle them with salt and eat them by themselves.
    - Portion the julienne zucchini and yellow squash into 1- or 2-cup portions that I can top with the Ground Meat Fra

Diavolo and steam in the microwave when I'm ready to eat!

- By now the egg cups should be done. Yay!
- Now increase the temperature to 425 degrees. Bake the chicken breast (20 minutes) and Brussels sprouts (30-40 minutes or until brown).

- Onto the organic strawberries.
  - Remove the stem and cut them in half for easier eating. I also store them in recycled Whole Foods containers.
- Next: **Not-Your-Everyday Chicken Salad** (Ingredients: 3 cans of organic canned chicken, 2 avocados, celery, green onion, lemon juice). Chicken salad lettuce wraps are my favorite! Boston lettuce works well in place of bread/tortillas.
  - Slice, then chop the celery and the green onion.
  - Drain the 3 cans of chicken and dump it into a glass bowl.
  - Cut the avocados in half and remove the pits....
  - Then scoop them into a separate bowl, add lemon juice and mash them with a fork (great substitute for mayo!)
  - Add salt and pepper to taste.
  - Add the mashed avocado to the chicken and mix with a spoon.
  - Fold in the green onions and celery.
  - Portion out ½ cup servings into plastic Ziploc containers.
- Portion a handful of each to a small/single serving plastic container for easy snacking: sliced peppers, sugar snap peas, baby carrots, etc. I like to recycle containers I get from Whole Foods.

- A handful of canned black olives is a great "fat" option. The only ingredients should be "olives" and (maybe) "salt."
- The Ground Meat Fra Diavolo should be cool enough to portion into containers... It's easy to go overboard so I use a food scale to weigh out 4-ish ounce portions.
- The baked chicken breast should also be done. I slice the chicken and, again, I use a food scale to weigh out 3 ounce portions into containers.
- When the Brussels sprouts are done, portion them out into larger plastic containers.
- I portion out **walnuts and/or macadamias** for some healthy fat (Walnuts and macadamias have the ideal 2:1 ratio of Omega 6: Omega 3)
- When the egg cups are cooled I portion them into Ziploc bags or containers. The perfect "to-go" breakfast!
- Done! 3:16pm. Total time: 62 minutes. The Mahaneys are ready for the week!
  - Put everything into the fridge! It's convenient and easy to get to when I need it. In the morning, when I leave for work, I just grab everything I need for the entire day, throw in in my cooler with an ice block and go!
  - I clean up - wash the pots & pans, throw the cutting board, knife & measuring cups into the dishwasher and I'm finished! All of my meals are prepared & portioned out for the next 3 days!

To see a video of my Weekly Food Prep please visit:
http://www.transformcrossfit.com/traceys_blog/weekly-food-prep.html

Paleo On-the-Go

PROTEIN

- Organic, pastured hard boiled eggs cooked beforehand
- Cold (leftover) organic, pastured chicken breast
- Cold (leftover) grass-fed London broil
- Nitrate-free organic sliced turkey breast
- Smoked wild salmon
- Tuna (Buy the kind that comes in a bag and it doesn't even need draining!)
- Sardines (Some people like 'em!)
- Jerky (nitrate-, nitrite-, and sugar-free) check out Steve's Paleo Goods PaleoJerky (https://www.stevespaleogoods.com/) or make your own!

CARBS

- Fresh fruit
- Pre-cut raw vegetables: broccoli, cauliflower, peppers, celery & carrot sticks, with salsa for dipping (check the ingredients for sugar!)

FAT

- Avocado
- Guacamole (check the ingredients to be sure it's Paleo-friendly)
- Canned olives (ingredients: olives, water & salt)
- Nuts & seeds (raw or dry roasted, salt optional)
- Coconut flakes

Dining Out

Divide your plate into three equal parts. On one-third of your plate put a lean protein no bigger or thicker than your palm. That's about three ounces for women and four ounces for men. Fill the other two-thirds with a variety of non-starchy vegetables (and a variety of colors). Add a dash of fat such as olive oil, avocado, walnuts, etc. The longer you adhere to strict weighing and measuring the more familiar you become with portion sizes and you will have an easier time "eyeballing" it. Especially if it's a food you eat often.

Obviously if you are preparing your own meals you know exactly what's going into them and your food log entries will be more accurate. The best thing you can do if you are trying to be strict (especially 100% paleo) is to not eat out… but that may not be realistic for you.

Some other tips:

- Get a main dish that is not a starch-based food. Try to choose the leanest meat or seafood available, cooked in a simple manner—by baking, broiling, sautéing, roasting, poaching, or steaming—without added starches and fats.

- Instead of a pasta dish, order a variety of vegetables served over a mound of spinach (sautéed in oil, not butter!) Have a small serving of fresh fruit for dessert.
- Ask the server to NOT bring the bread basket!
- Keep the meal as simple as you can; the fewer ingredients, the better. Don't be afraid to special order something that is not on the menu. Restaurants nowadays are typically pretty accommodating. If all else fails, mention that you have food allergies (which may actually be accurate!)
- Make your own paleo-friendly dressing and bring it with you.
- Check out the restaurant's menu on their website (or contact them directly) and know what your options are before you arrive.

Traveling

- Dining out (see above)
- Buying food and taking it with you in a cooler (see above)
- Buying food in supermarkets, grocery stores, and even roadside markets along the way (Fresh fruit & veggies are always available!)
- Carry with you for emergencies: Steve's Paleo Goods (https://www.stevespaleogoods.com/)

Step 14 –
3...2...1...GO!

What to expect during 28+ days of 100% Paleo

WEEK ONE

Biggest Changes

- Putting different kinds of food into your body
- Getting accustomed to preparing new meals
- Getting accustomed to unfamiliar routines of how, where, and maybe with whom you eat

Tips

- Stay strong! Tape your *"Describe Your Objective"* (from Step Five) to the fridge for when you need a reminder of why you are doing this.
- Be prepared! Keep enough food on-hand.
- If you are hungry EAT!
- Your body is still adjusting to using fat for energy instead of carbs (hence the low energy). Be sure to get enough lean protein and healthy fat!
- Get plenty of rest. Relax. Take a hot bath, read a book, or watch something funny.
- Have a sense of humor and acceptance.

- Don't focus on what you are giving up… Instead focus on everything you have to gain: a lean and healthy body, vibrant health, and a long life.
- Have a "go-to" approved food option for when sugar cravings arise… Whether it's bacon, almond butter, coconut flakes… Just don't go crazy. Too much of anything (even if it's paleo) is not okay.
- Practice mindful eating.
- Instead of alcohol, enjoy a cup of herbal tea or a glass of Kombucha.
- Reach out to a supportive friend or loved one.
- **If you "fall off the wagon" get back on track immediately at your next meal or snack (back to Day One). Don't waste energy worrying and let go of judgment toward yourself. Recommit.**

DAYS 1-2

What you might be feeling:
- Good, Motivated

What you might be thinking:
- "This isn't so bad. I got this!"
- "Why do people think this is so hard?"

DAYS 3-5

What you might be experiencing:
- Possible withdrawal symptoms from sugars, caffeine, chemicals in foods: headaches, irritability, changes in mood, fatigue, low blood sugar

- Cravings... They will go away!!! Fight through it. Make sure you are eating enough.

What you might be feeling:

- Mentally: Still excited and motivated.
- Physically: Low energy.

DAY 6

What you might be feeling:

- Grumpy and irritable.
- Ready to quit. DON'T!

DAY 7

What you might be feeling:

- Empowered and excited! You made it through a week!
- Lighter and cleaner.

What you might be experiencing:

- Clearing of sinuses.

WEEK TWO

DAY 8

What you might be feeling:

- Overwhelmed. But you made it through your first weekend! Be sure to plan your meals for the week and have plenty of food on hand.

What you might be thinking:

- "What's the point?" Pull out that *Describe Your Objective* as a reminder!

<u>DAYS 9 – 10</u>

What you might be feeling:

- "This is too much" or "I don't have time for this!" Remember that every choice you make is moving you closer to or further from your goals. It's a daily choice to eat healthy and PERSERVERE! You can do this!

What you might be experiencing:

- Clearer, brighter skin
- Reduced indigestion, heartburn and acid stomach

<u>DAY 11</u>

What you might be feeling:

- Pretty good... You are almost halfway there! But don't let that be an excuse to go off-plan!

What you might be experiencing:

- Increased energy levels
- Less stiffness of joints

<u>DAYS 12-13</u>

What you might be feeling:

- "Hangry" (hungry and angry). If you are hungry EAT! Remember, this isn't a diet... It's a way of life!
- Losing motivation? Focus on all of the good changes that are taking place in your mood, sleep habits, appearance, athletic performance!

What you might be experiencing:

- Normalization of bowel function

DAY 14

What you might be feeling:

- Excited!! You. Are. Awesome! You are halfway there! Keep your eyes on the prize. You can do this!

WEEK THREE

DAYS 15-17

What you might be experiencing:

- Excited! You are over the hump!

What you might be feeling:

- Proud! You should! Stay focused and on track. And remember to always be prepared with food on hand!

DAY 18

- You are almost there. You have come so far. Think about all the positive changes you have made and how it has affected your life.

DAYS 19-21

What you might be thinking:

- "When the heck is this going to be over?!" Remember that it's a marathon, not a sprint. You may be tackling some issues with food that you have had for years... You may not be able to "fix" everything in only three weeks. Be patient and kind with yourself.

WEEK FOUR

DAY 22-26

What you might be feeling:

- Nervous… about reintroducing off-plan foods next week. Are you feeling so good you don't want to lose it? First off, you don't *have to* do anything. If you want to continue eating this way, by all means, do so. But if you want to *truly* know what foods may be having a negative effect on how you look, feel and perform, it's a good idea to reintroduce them at some point and see what happens.

DAY 27

- **One more day**! You may be feeling anxious about your reintroduction. No matter what happens, get rid of the black-and-white, all-or-nothing thinking. Remember you always have a choice.

DAY 28

- When these 24 hours are up you will be victorious!! Congratulations!

Remember that the period of time you spend at this level will vary depending on your weight-loss goals and your current state of health. It may take only a few weeks to alter blood sugar, cholesterol, triglycerides, or blood pressure, for example, but it could take several months to lose a substantial amount of weight. Maybe you need 28 days, three months, six months, or more. If that's the case STAY WITH

IT! It only gets better! Once you have completed this stage you will complete seven days of reintroduction (I'll talk about this in Step Fifteen – Reintroduction). After completing your reintroduction you may move to Level Two for maintenance (except for those with chronic disease, who may do better with long-term adherence to strict paleo). You can always return to Level One in the future anytime you feel you have gotten off track.

Step 15 – Reintroduction

But FIRST... Let's conduct another Wellness Audit

Be sure to complete this BEFORE you begin your Reintroduction!

Answer the questions on this list with the numbers: 0, 1, 2 or 3.

0 = Frequently, 1 = Sometimes, 2 = Rarely, 3 = Never

1. _Do you experience headaches?_

2. _Do you tend to get a cold and/or virus each year?_

3. _Do you have bowel movements less than several times per day?_

4. _Do you experience constipation?_

5. _Do you experience diarrhea?_

6. _Do you experience pain and/or stiffness in your joints or muscles?_

7. _Do you experience itchy and/or watery eyes and nose at certain times of year?_

8. _Do you experience congestion or mucus in your throat?_

9. _Do you get bloated after eating?_

10. _Do you have extra body fat that you cannot seem to lose with exercise and/or diet?_

11. _Do you experience indigestion heartburn, gas, and/or acid stomach?_

12. _Do you have bad breath?_

13. _Do you have body odor?_

14. _Do you crave certain foods, especially starchy, sugary foods?_

15. *Do you have a skin condition such as itchy skin or pimples?*

16. *Do you have low energy levels?*

17. *Do you rely heavily on caffeine for energy?*

18. *Do you experience restless sleep and/or insomnia?*

19. *Do you experience bad moods, sadness, or depression?*

Now add up all of the numbers to figure out your score and compare it to your score when you began.

"After/In Progress" Photos and Measurements

1. Take another photo of yourself (using a cell phone camera is fine) wearing as little as possible. Compare it to your "before photo."

2. Using a tape measure, take and record the following measurements and compare them to your measurements when you began:

    - Your hips at the widest part (be sure to keep the tape level).
    - Your waist at the belly button (*not* the narrowest part).

Reintroduction

Days 29 – 35

On day 29, introduce ONE type of food from the "What to Avoid" list (Step Ten – Go Paleo!) into your daily meals. A moderate serving will do. Observe, feel, and record what happens over the next 24-48 hours. Repeat on days 31, 33 and 35.

This is the part where the wheels usually fall off the bus…. but it is SO crucial. If you are anything like me you have been dreaming of all of the things you plan to eat the minute the elimination phase is over. Not so fast. We don't want to open up the flood gates and within five days have you right back where you started (and feeling like crap)! This defeats the whole purpose of what we are trying to accomplish! Remember: The only way to figure out what an optimal diet for you looks like is to **experiment and observe**.

Every 48 hours for one week (days 29, 31, 33 and 35) you will add back those foods that you have eliminated **one-by-one** (experiment) and see how you respond (observe). You ***will continue to follow your strict paleo plan except for that one item.*** Any noticeable change in your physical or mental experience is an indication that you might be sensitive or fully allergic to that food!).

o   <u>Day 29 </u>– Eat ONE non-paleo item (i.e. milk)

o   <u>Day 31</u> – Eat ONE non-paleo item (i.e. non-gluten-containing grain such as oatmeal or quinoa)

o   <u>Day 33</u> – Eat ONE non-paleo item (i.e. legumes / soy)

o   <u>Day 35</u> – Eat ONE non-paleo item (i.e. gluten-containing grain such as bread)

For each item you reintroduce, record the following information:

- *Date and time*
- *Food*
- *Amount*
- *How do you feel immediately after eating it?*
- *What are you feeling in your belly?*
- *Shortly after you eat it, do you experience a runny nose, bloating, fatigue, headache, mucus in your throat?*
- *How are your energy levels one hour after eating?*

- *How are your bowel movements the next day? Are they the same/as frequent as they were days 1-28? If not, how are they different?*
- *How does your skin look?*
- *How do you feel emotionally/mentally?*
- *How did you sleep after eating it?*
- *Provide any additional information you feel is relevant.*

After completing your reintroduction you may move to Level Two for maintenance (except for those with chronic disease, who may do better with long-term adherence to strict paleo). You can always return to Level One in the future anytime you feel you have gotten off track. Check out the next chapter (Step Sixteen – Maintaining Your New Body) for tips on relapse prevention and recovery plans.

Step 16 –
Maintaining Your New Body

We have done several paleo/nutrition Challenges at our gym since we opened our doors in 2009, each lasting between 28 and 40 days. The **goal** was for participants to follow a strict paleo diet (no grains, processed foods, legumes, dairy products, or sugar) for the length of the challenge. The **purpose** was for participants to not just clean up their diets, but also to determine what foods they were sensitive to.

Everyone who participated saw phenomenal results. On day the last day of the Challenge they were looking, feeling, and performing better than they had been on day one - possibly better than they had in their entire life! At the end of the challenge, participants were encouraged (if they chose) to *slowly* reintroduce small portions of non-paleo foods (one by one) to see what happened. They knew almost immediately which foods they were sensitive to because of how bad they felt (physically). Sadly, the day after the Challenge ended, many (not all) of the athletes who participated had *completely* fallen off the wagon and within a *week* were "enjoying" all of the foods that were "off limits" for 28+ days! The flood gates opened and within three months those very athletes were approaching me saying, "You guys need to have another Paleo Challenge!" Where is the good in that?!

By now you should have a pretty good awareness based on your Reintroduction Assessments of exactly what foods are having a negative impact on your health and wellness. Based on what you know to be true you can now *choose* how often you include those foods as part of your regular eating plan, if at all.

Just know that it won't always be easy. You will struggle from time to time. Everyone struggles. It's normal. You are human. The sooner you embrace that and cope with it the happier you will be. You have proven that you have the coping skills and behavior change strategies needed to cope with it, get control, and get back on track quickly.

Relapse prevention

- **Never be hungry.** If you let yourself get too hungry you are more likely to binge and/or make poor food choices.
- **Eating must be pleasurable and functional.** There is no reason to survive on baked chicken and steamed broccoli (unless of course you love baked chicken and steamed broccoli). Experiment with new recipes. Make Google your new best friend!
- **Keep a detailed food log of everything you eat.** Food logs work by increasing accountability and awareness. Remember the B.L.T. Rule: If you bite it, lick it, or taste it, it gets recorded.
- **Focus on what has worked for you up to now and stick with that.** If it ain't broke why fix it?
- **Predetermine your "treats" ahead of time.** Decide what, when, and how often. Figure out what works for you and what doesn't. And make it worth it! (also see "Treat Guide" below)

- **Decide in advance.** Anticipate occasions where you will be faced with temptation and be prepared with a plan.
- **Plan ahead and be prepared.** Planning and preparation are crucial when it comes to good nutrition. You should always know what, when, and where your next meal will be.
- **Avoid your triggers.** If having it in your house makes it too tempting to avoid, get it out of your house! Out of sight, out of mind.
- **Focus on portion size.** If you mindlessly put food on your plate with no attention to portion size you are more likely to eat more just because it's in front of you. If you weigh and measure your portions you may be surprised to find that you don't need as much as you think you do.
- **Think long-term and be realistic.** It's a marathon, not a sprint. Your long-term eating plan needs to be sustainable whether you are at home, dining out, at work, on the road, or on an airplane. The word "diet" comes from the ancient Greek root which means "way of life." It's not to be thought of as simply a short-term period of hunger and deprivation just to fit into a swimsuit.
- **Set some hard, fast rules.** Know *how* you are going to eat each day and *why*. Plan out in advance what an awesome (clean) day of eating will look like. Make a commitment to adhere to your rules no matter what.

No one can be 100 percent Paleo 100 percent of the time, nor should they be. I encourage you predetermine your "treats" ahead of time. Decide right now, in advance. Will you allow yourself three treats per week? Two treats? One treat per week? Will your treats occur on the same day each week or will the days vary based on your agenda? Or will you strive for 100 percent compliance until a treat crosses your path that is really worth eating? Set a goal, write it down and commit to it. Continue to keep a food log and pay close attention to the affect each food has on your progress. You will figure out what you can and cannot get away with. Reassess monthly and make changes as needed.

Notice I said treat and not cheat. The word cheat has a negative connotation. Saying you cheated implies that you have done something bad. A treat is something that you allow yourself to indulge in from time to time without guilt because it's delicious and pleasurable.

A Treat Guide...

- **Make it special.** How often do we (over)eat food that doesn't even taste good or satisfy us? Don't eat something just because it's in front of you. If you are going stray from your plan, for crying out loud, make it worth it!

- **Commit to your predetermined treat days.** If I commit to two treats per week and I choose ahead of time that I will enjoy one treat on Tuesday and one treat on Friday... and then someone shows up with a container of homemade chocolate peanut butter buckeyes on Thursday, I *do not* give myself the option of eating one. If they are still available on Friday (maybe) I will eat one then. Just because a treat presents itself unexpectedly that is not permission to get off course!

- **Travel to get it.** If I am really craving a chocolate chip cookie I don't want just any old cookie. I want a Starbucks chocolate chunk cookie. It just so happens that there is a Starbucks one-half mile from where we live. So, since I don't keep junk food in the house, I head over to Starbucks and buy one – only if it's my predetermined treat day, of course. If I have to travel to a destination to get the cookie it makes it even more special.

- **Know your triggers.** Don't indulge in something that has the potential to trigger an all-out binge. If you are craving pizza but you know you won't stop until you've devoured the entire pie, pizza is probably not the best choice for you.

- **Write it down.** Record your treats in your food log just as you would any other food. Even better, write down specifically what you plan to eat *before* you eat it. At our favorite restaurant they have a chocolate flourless cake on the dessert menu that I absolutely love. I decide ahead of time that I will share a slice with Andy... Sometimes I'll take it a step further and commit to how many bites I will have. When we are through with dinner, and the server presents the dessert menu, I don't give myself the option of ordering a separate dessert for myself or eating more than the predetermined amount. I usually find that I am satisfied with less than I want.

- **Serving size.** Ideally a treat should be a *single* serving of one (or two) off-plan item(s). Common sense should tell you that if you eat a half gallon if ice cream in one sitting it qualifies as a full-out binge. If I am going out to dinner and I want a treat I will order, say, a hamburger (hold the cheese and the bun) with a side of fries (treat = fries). Or, if I want to eat the bun I'll sub a salad for the fries (treat = bun). Or, if I want dessert I'll have a piece of lean protein and a salad for dinner and I'll split the dessert with someone (treat = ½ dessert). For more on serving size, check out "Avoid food bombs," below.

- **Portion it out.** Avoid foods in bulk form. If I decide on tortilla chips and guacamole I need it to be portioned out otherwise I will continue to eat until the entire bag of chips is gone… and I will probably lick the bowl of guacamole clean. Seriously. I will. The solution for me is to pour *one serving* of chips into a bowl and I do the same with the guacamole. The idea is to enjoy the treat without going overboard.

- **Don't eat mindlessly.** Don't pull out a pint of ice cream and plop yourself in front of the television (or computer). When you are enjoying a treat ENJOY IT for goodness sake! Why distract yourself from something so delicious!?

- **Avoid food bombs.** Any food (or meal) that contains grains *and* gluten *and* dairy *and* sugar (or any other combination of off-plan items) can be considered a food bomb (think Thanksgiving dinner). Some examples include: a cheeseburger and fries with ketchup (grains, gluten, dairy, potatoes and sugar), pizza (grains, gluten and dairy), a Brownie a la Mode (grains, gluten, dairy and sugar), loaded nachos (corn/grains, dairy, legumes, and God knows what else). A food bomb will probably leave you feeling like… well, like a bomb went off in your gut, and will likely take longer to recover from. Now I realize this may not always be easy since most delicious treats contain more than one off-plan item. But do the best you can.

- **Space out your treats.** Try to space out your treats over the course of a week. This will have less of an impact on your insulin levels and will be much easier to recover from. Spacing your treats too close together (i.e. dinner on Friday and brunch on Saturday) could potentially take days to recover from and make it that much more difficult to get back on track.

- **Remember, you *always* have a choice.** You are never obligated to eat anything you don't want to eat. Whether you are at a holiday party, a business dinner, or a friend's house for lunch, you are never obligated to eat something just because it's there or because it's offered to you. If you decide *in advance* that it will count as one of your treats for the week that is your choice. But you *always* have a choice. If are out with a group of friends and everyone lights up a cigarette, would you smoke one if it was offered to you even though you are a non-smoker? Of course not! The same applies to your food choices. It's not rude to politely say "no thank you" to something that you don't want to eat, especially if it's something that you know makes you sick! Anyone who cares about you will understand and respect that.

What to do when you get off track (and you will)...

There will be occasions when you will make extremely poor food choices and/or you will eat more than you should. You may relapse into old, familiar, ineffective and destructive habits that hinder your progress. The difference now is that it should happen much less frequently. But when it does happen you will need to be ready with a plan to help you recover quickly. Use the skills you have learned (that maybe you didn't possess before) to minimize the damage and get back on track.

When a relapse occurs...

You could...

a) Roll around in guilt and remorse and berate yourself for your "failure" for the next seven days (or more). But that would be very unhealthy and unproductive and would likely lead to a vicious cycle of emotional eating.

b) Let it completely derail you from your long-term plan. Let's call it the "Fu@k it" effect: the line of thinking that says once you cheat you've blown it so you might as well binge. But that black-and-white thinking would only leave you feeling crappy longer, which will make it that much harder to get back on track.

c) Understand that it's all part of the process. Pause and ask yourself, "How can I learn from this? What can I do differently next time?" Accept that you got off course, learn from it, and move on to your Recovery Plan IMMEDIATELY.

Which option will YOU choose? (Correct answer: Option 'c')

DOs and DON'Ts

Do NOT rationalize or justify your actions.

Instead:

- Recognize that you had a setback and move on.
- Hold yourself accountable for behavior that is not in line with what you want to achieve.
- Be honest with yourself about the fact that you failed. Take ownership for it and analyze what went wrong.
- Engage in solving the problem and finding a solution.
- Move on to your Recovery Plan immediately.

Do NOT say to yourself:

- *"It could have been worse."*

   Of course it could have. But it also could have been better.

- *"I had a really tough workout today so I can eat this."*

   You cannot out-exercise a poor diet. Most people overestimate the number of calories they actually burn during a workout. Even if you could burn off all of the calories consumed during a binge, a workout will not undo the resulting inflammation and gut irritation. Besides, everyone knows that "abs are made in the kitchen, not the gym!"

- *"Life's too short! You only live once."*

   That is true. But do you want to just survive.... or do you want to THRIVE?! This is the only body you will ever have in this lifetime. Wouldn't you rather do whatever you can to make it the healthiest body possible?

- *"I'm doing better than I was before."*

   That's awesome but it's a slippery slope! It's those kinds of rationalizations that will get you back to square one before you know it. Remember: You are never standing still. <u>Every</u> choice you make is either moving you closer to or *further from* your goals – and optimal wellness. Practice saying, "I am going to strive to be even better today than I was yesterday and better tomorrow than I am today!"

Do NOT set a date in the future to get back on track.

- Do it right NOW! Otherwise you will find yourself buying time while you rationalize why you shouldn't get back on track.
- Just because you fall off the wagon on Thursday does not mean you have to wait until the following Monday to get back on track (that goes for all of you Type A personalities out there!)
- The quicker you diagnose your failures by identifying specific behaviors that did or did not happen, the more successful you will be at maintaining your new body.

Have a Plan of Recovery

When I make poor food choices I feel crappy. When I feel crappy I default towards foods that are fatty, salty, greasy, sugary... *aaaand* not so healthy. So I need to decide *before* the failure occurs (and I'm feeling crappy and emotional) how I will handle it when it happens. That means having a Recovery Plan mapped out (and written down) ahead of time. The goal is to interrupt the pattern as quickly as possible. As Dr. Barry Sears says, "you are only as good as your next meal." You should know *in advance* exactly what your next meal and all remaining meals will look like. Follow it up with a full day of meals that are in line with your healthy eating philosophy and you will be feeling good again before you know it. (I think it goes without saying, but starving yourself or over-exercising in an attempt to compensate for overindulging is not the solution. It's unhealthy and counterproductive and will only set you up for a binge later. The same goes for purging, abusing laxatives, or any other attempt to get rid of what you consumed).

When in recovery mode I try to keep my meals relatively low in carbohydrates to get my blood sugar/insulin levels back to a normal range. This means emphasizing lean protein (poultry, fish, lean beef, eggs/egg whites), vegetables (especially greens) and healthy fats, and avoiding fruits, starchy vegetables and sugars. Here is an example of what a Recovery Day looks like for me:

- *Upon rising:* I keep a gallon of room temperature distilled water (with a splash of lemon juice added) next to my bed.* As soon as my feet hit the floor I take ten to twenty large gulps. (You can warm it in the microwave if you prefer). Then I head to the kitchen and brew a single cup of coffee. While the coffee is brewing I take two teaspoons of fish oil (with a splash of unsweetened almond milk) for its anti-inflammatory properties.

- *Exercise:* Running helps to get the blood and endorphins flowing. This is a good time for me to pray, meditate and get my head straight. I vary the duration and intensity based on my mood. Sometimes I do several short (100-400 meters) or long (800+ meters) high-intensity intervals with a few minutes rest in between. At other times I go for a longer, lower intensity run.

- *Breakfast:* One whole pastured egg + four egg whites scrambled with non-starchy vegetables (spinach, mushrooms, peppers, tomatoes, onions, etc.), one-quarter to one-half an avocado, black coffee with a dash of cinnamon and stevia.

- *Snack:* One or two slices of Applegate Farms organic/natural turkey breast, one or two handfuls of raw sliced vegetables (red peppers, cucumbers, carrots and sugar snap peas are my favorites), six to nine raw almonds or a small closed handful of olives.

- *Lunch:* Three to four ounces of chicken breast (or some other lean protein) with a large mixed salad (spring mix, spinach, arugula, peppers, tomatoes, cucumbers, avocado, walnuts and homemade balsamic dressing), eight ounces of Kombucha.

- *Dinner:* Three to four ounces of organic lean protein (chicken, pork, fish or grass-fed beef), a heaping portion of steamed or roasted non-starchy vegetables (broccoli, zucchini, Brussels sprouts, spinach) drizzled with olive oil.

- *Dessert:* One-half to one cup of fresh berries sprinkled with cinnamon.

- *Before bed:* Two teaspoons of "Natural Calm" (magnesium supplement) in hot water.

- *I make it my goal to drink eight to twelve eight-ounce glasses of water throughout the day (between meals).

You may also consider spending a few days (or more) back at Level One (100% Paleo) to allow your body to get back with the program, get yourself fit, and then move on to Level One (The Open-Meal Approach).

TESTIMONIALS

Caitlyn from Pennington, NJ

If I had to sum up a paleo lifestyle into one word, I would use the word relief. It has given me relief from migraines and allergies, a relief from chasing numbers on a scale, a relief to counting endless calories. Before following Paleo I was in a constant battle of disordered eating and endless cardio and hours at the gym.

I grew up eating the standard American diet which caused me to be very overweight as a young child. I always remember the doctors lecturing my parents about my weight, but it never bothered me. I was active, and in my mind healthy; just stuck with big bones and a slow metabolism. One day going into my sophomore year of college I woke up and decided I would make a change. It started out with the best of intentions, cutting out bad foods and exercising more. This quickly changed and I was cutting out more and more foods. I was able to drop my weight about half in six months, going from 185 to around 95-100lbs.

I eventually was able to get back to a "healthy" weight but never felt healthy or happy with myself. I was still constantly struggling with eating "normal" and making up for what I ate at the gym. When I began CrossFit I knew a little about paleo, but thought it was too difficult for me to ever maintain. I joined in a paleo challenge which I was initially only trying to look my best for an upcoming wedding. I decided to dive in and commit 100% for one month.

As we began the challenge I took a picture and was okay with how I looked. Not thrilled, but thought it was the best I could do. Two weeks into living paleo I was shocked at the new picture I took. My stomach was flat and I felt great. I could sleep through the night, and have plenty of energy for the next day. Although, I did not eat many grains before paleo they definitely had an effect on my body, making me puffy and bloated. This second week I also had a breakthrough in how I felt towards food. I finally was enjoying what I ate and was full and satisfied. My CrossFit workouts were becoming easier and my bad habit of smoking was beginning to become less and less appealing. Over a year later I still follow a paleo lifestyle and couldn't be happier. My monthly migraines subsided, and my allergies that I received shots for as a child disappeared. I now eat lots of various meats (I only would allow chicken or turkey before) and healthy fats(bacon!)and I am not afraid if I "cheat" every now and then on something like chocolate. I enjoy the food and brush it off and start fresh the next day. I will make sure that my "cheat" is still grain free. Grains I noticed give me a terrible food hangover, and takes me days to really recover.

I do not measure my food. I eat when I'm hungry and stop when I'm full. I usually begin my day with two egg cups and 3 slices of bacon. For lunch I eat a mixture of leftovers from the night before. A favorite is ground turkey with Brussels sprouts and sweet potatoes with a side of guacamole and baby carrots. When I get home I'll have a handful of fruit and nuts and then dinner. I will cook a protein with seasonal vegetables using coconut oil, or grass-fed butter. I never considered paleo as a diet, but a healthy lifestyle that has healed me inside and out. I don't really look at the scale, I use the mirror and my clothes as my guide. I am stronger than I ever realized I could be. I can run farther and faster than I ever imagined. (I could barely run a mile in high school). This year not only did I run my fastest mile, but ran a 10 mile race in 1:45. I am excited when I look and see new muscles forming especially my abs. Although I am not the same weight as I was at my smallest, some clothes fit me just as well now if not better than before.

Cathy from Pennington, New Jersey

Q: What were your goals when you were first introduced to the paleo diet?

I primarily wanted to lose weight. At the time I had a 4 and 6 year old and I never lost that baby weight. I had at least 20 lbs. to lose. But I was also interested in eating healthier. For most of my life, I never concerned myself with what types of foods I ate. Food was a form of entertainment and I ate whatever I wanted. Up until I got pregnant I was always somewhat thin so I never really worried about it. After having kids, I realized I had to start worrying about it! I was about to turn 40 when I started eating paleo and I couldn't get away with my unhealthy diet anymore.

Q: How long have you been following a paleo way of eating?

I have been eating paleo for just over 2 years now.

Q: Do you weigh yourself?

I used to weigh myself daily but I rarely weigh myself anymore. I focus on how my body looks and how my clothes fit.

Q: What kind of results have you seen (i.e. body composition, athletic performance, etc.)? Please be sure to include things that the scale can't measure! Such as: How has going paleo affected your energy levels, appearance, bodily functions, mood, outlook, sleep, symptoms/conditions, etc.?

I started eating paleo and working out at a CrossFit gym in September, 2011. By mid-January, 2012, I lost 3 inches in my waist, 2 inches in my chest, 2.5 inches in my hips and 1.5 inches in my thighs. I also had lost 13 pounds! In 3 months, that is pretty good results. I really couldn't believe how the inches were melting off of me. And I felt better! I had way more energy. I ate so many bad carbs before – cereals, granola bars, pretzels, crackers, etc. that caused my energy level to spike up and down dramatically. I felt less hungry and more even-keeled.

By July, 2012, I had lost 6.5 inches in my waist, 5 inches in my hips and 4 inches in my thighs. And I had lost 21 pounds. By October, I had lost 24 pounds! That was my lowest weight since my 20's. I was very strict paleo but still had my wine and occasional cheats. But when I would splurge on that amazing wood-fired pizza at the local joint, I would feel so lethargic and bloated for several days. I feel like by eating a paleo diet, my body changed to the weight and proportions it was supposed to be without all of the extra flab.

Q: What have you done in the past (pre-paleo) to try to achieve your goals?

Before getting married, both my husband and I did the Atkin's diet and had success. However, it just didn't feel like a healthy way to eat and it wasn't a diet I could maintain indefinitely. We did lost weight though. Other than that, I rarely dieted. But I was probably what you could have called "skinny-fat", especially in my 30's. I was not at all toned but have always been a size 4 until having kids.

Q: Do you still struggle? If so, what do you struggle with?

I struggle most around the holidays when there are so many "bad" foods at parties and gatherings. I love cheese and crackers, chips and dip and all kinds of savory snacks. They are hard to resist for me. I also love to drink wine and often have more than I should! But I usually give myself some leeway to be bad at these times and I get back on the wagon in January!

Q: How do you handle cravings? What do you do?

I try to find an acceptable paleo alternative to what I am craving. I often crave salty snacks so I will grab a handful of salted nuts instead. Or if I have a sweet tooth, I will eat a clementine or an apple. Though I really want a candy bar, I know I will regret that too much if I eat it. Eating some fruit really satisfies that sweet craving and I no longer want candy or cookies.

Q: What was your initial approach to paleo? Did you jump right in to 100%? One-meal-at-a time approach? Open Meal approach?

I started at 100% paleo (with the occasional glass of wine!). I also really incorporated the Zone diet after a few months. That really helps with balancing your meals and snacks and making you feel more satisfied. I was very strict with myself, especially for the first year. I *liked having clear-cut rules to follow. And the results I was seeing was a continual motivating factor to keep at it!*

Q: What changes did you make at home when you went paleo (i.e. Did you clean out your cabinets/pantry/fridge? If so, what did you toss? How did your family meals change?)

I have small children so I had to keep all of the snacky, sugary stuff, unfortunately. However, I usually have the discipline to steer clear. I try to modify the kids' diets too. I rarely feed them pasta and our dinners consist of a meat and several vegetables most nights. They are fine with it and are gradually becoming more educated about eating healthy, "real" foods as opposed to the processed garbage.

Q: Was/is your family on-board with the paleo way of eating? Please explain.

My husband was initially pretty skeptical about the paleo diet. Having done Atkin's before, he was always in support of a lower-carb diet though. So he continued eating his Nature Valley granola bar every morning and his fruit and cottage cheese for lunch almost every day. For dinner, he would have a protein with several vegetables. Even when he was just eating a paleo dinner every night (non-paleo during the day), he lost a few pounds from that! Mark had a physical around the time I began eating paleo and realized that he had slightly high cholesterol and high blood sugar. They recommended he go on a low-dose of Lipitor. He wanted to change his diet and see if he got results. He could see paleo was working for me, as I had already lost over 10 pounds, but he wanted to do the research himself. He read The Paleo

Solution by Robb Wolf in the summer of 2012. It made sense to him and he jumped on the paleo bandwagon 100%.

Mark didn't exercise at all, nor had he done much exercising in his entire adult life. His daily exercise consisted of the mile or so walk from Penn Station to his office near Grand Central Station every morning and evening. Within about 3-4 months, he had lost 23 pounds. He has always been a slim man but now he was back to what he weighed in his 20's. His waist size is back to what it was in college and he is now 45 years old.

Both Mark and I take no pills or vitamins, aside from the occasional Advil as needed. We both had physicals this fall and we are both healthy with blood work in normal to above-average range. (I can give numbers if you need them.)

It is also very interesting that prior to eating paleo, Mark experienced heartburn regularly. He would take Zantac daily but he still suffered with it. Nothing helped. He also would occasionally get inexplicable rashes around his ankles and calves. Our primary care doctor sent him to an infectious disease specialist and that doctor thought he might have some sort of auto immune disorder and wanted to do all sorts of tests on him. Mark never followed up with any of that. However, he **never** gets heartburn except for the occasional cheat meals we have, such as going out for pizza. It wasn't the spiciness or tomato-based foods that were bothering him at all, as we always assumed. It was clearly the gluten in the pasta and pizza! And he has never gotten one of those crazy, itchy rashes again since switching to a paleo diet. So Mark definitely learned that he does have a sort of gluten intolerance, though he has never been formally tested for it.

Q: How do you deal with people who are unsupportive?

My parents, despite the fact we have been eating this way for over 2 years now, refuse to acknowledge that this might be a healthier way to eat and live. My dad has severe Type-2 diabetes and the paleo way of eating would benefit him immensely. My mom has high cholesterol and the diet would probably reverse that if she tried. Both are overweight. But they are both of the old-school mentality that pills and prescriptions will fix all of their problems and enable their unhealthy habits. It's very frustrating to watch but you can teach old dogs new tricks in some cases.

Q: Did you keep a food log? Are you keeping one now? If so, how has it helped you? (Please include a sample of an entry)

No, though I should, I don't typically keep a food log (unless we were doing at paleo challenge at tCF).

Q: What does a typical day look like for you in terms of nutrition (Please be as specific as possible) starting with when you wake up.

- *Breakfast: 2 cups of coffee (with half and half and a little agave nectar), a few slices of deli ham or some sausage, Kit's Organic's bar or Larabar*
- *Lunch: Salad with grilled chicken, HB egg, tuna, salmon. Or the previous night's leftovers*
- *Mid-afternoon snack: HB egg or beef jerky (sugar free) with a piece of fruit or some carrots or other veggies, handful of nuts*
- *Dinner: Grilled meat with a large portion of veggies. Typically with some wine. ☺*

- *Lots of water, sparkling mineral water or iced tea throughout the day.*

Q: Do you have a plan each week for grocery shopping, meal planning, food prep, etc? If so, please explain.

I usually plan 3-4 days at a time. That's all I seem to be able to do! It's hard for me to buy a whole week's worth of meals. Since I don't work outside of the home, I have the ability to go to the store several times a week and cook a fresh meal every night without a problem.

LINKS & RESOURCES

BOOKS

Primal Body – Primal Mind | Beyond the Paleo Diet for Total Health and a Longer Life by Nora T. Gedgaudas

The Protein Power Lifeplan by Drs. Michael and Mary Dan Eades

The Paleo Diet (revised) by Dr. Loren Cordain

The Paleo Solution by Rob Wolff

The Primal Blueprint by Mark Sisson

Well Fed by Melissa Joulwan (cookbook)

It Starts With Food by Dallas & Melissa Hartwig

Clean by Dr. Alejandro Junger M.D.

WEBSITES

Primal Body Primal Mind | Beyond the Paleo Diet http://www.primalbody-primalmind.com/

Protein Power http://proteinpower.com/

The Paleo Diet http://thepaleodiet.com/

Robb Wolf http://robbwolf.com/

Chris Kresser http://chriskresser.com/

Mark's Daily Apple http://www.marksdailyapple.com/

Whole9 http://whole9life.com/

OTHER HELPFUL LINKS

How to eat a milk-free, wheat-free, soy-free, peanut-free diet
http://www.foodallergy.org/document.doc?id=133

Other Names for Sugar That Appear on Labels
http://www.fitsugar.com/Other-Names-Sugar-Appear-Labels-810571